CARDIOVASCULAR PRINCIPLES

A REGISTRY EXAM PREPARATION GUIDE

Terry Reynolds, BS, RDCS

School Of Cardiac & Vascular Ultrasound
Arizona Heart Foundation
Phoenix, Arizona

Dedicated to

My beloved youngest brother James Martin
who gave up too soon

Cardiovascular Principles — A Registry Exam Preparation Guide
Arizona Heart Foundation
1910 E. Thomas Road, Suite 100
Phoenix, AZ 85016
(602) 200-0437

ISBN 0-9635767-6-3

TABLE OF CONTENTS

Chapter 6 (Unit 6). Principles of Cardiac Hemodynamics

APPENDICES

IV

PREFACE

This cardiovascular principles guidebook represents three years of classroom registry examination presentations at the School of Cardiac Ultrasound. The apparent strength of the guide is that it takes the cardiovascular principles examination outline and breaks it down into its smallest components, discusses each component thoroughly, with each section followed by practice review and board review examination questions. The Cardiovascular Principles at a Glance section provides a condensation of the pertinent material, and the Cardiovascular Principles 500 section provides a challenging final test. When completed, the reader is confident that the cardiovascular principles portion of the registry examination has been carefully studied.

I would like to thank Edward B. Diethrich, M.D. for his strong support of ultrasound education; Mary Grace Warner, M.D. for her belief in me many years ago; Jack L. Dunham, Ph.D., who designed, edited, and provided focus for the manuscript; our clinical site instructors for their kindness extended to our students; and most importantly, to my students for their unbounded energy to know the reason why.

I offer this guidebook to you with the sincere hope that it will contribute to your continued success.

Terry Reynolds, BS, RDCS
Phoenix, Arizona

CARDIOVASCULAR PRINCIPLES TEST OUTLINE

I. Anatomy of the Heart   4% - 8%
    A. Chambers and Related Septa
    B. Valves and Related Apparatus
    C. Arterial-Venous System
    D. Conduction System
    E. Layers
    F. Relational Anatomy

II. Basic Embryology   1% - 3%
    A. Primitive Heart Tube
        1. Formation from primitive vascular tube
        2. Sinus venosus
        3. Cardiac loop
        4. Aortic arches
        5. Septation
        6. Valve formation
    B. Comparison of Fetal and Postnatal Circulation

III. Congenital Defects   1% - 3%
    A. Abnormalities of Septation
    B. Abnormal Vasculature and Resulting Lesions
    C. Persistence of Normal Fetal Communication
    D. Valvular Anomalies

IV. Cardiac Physiology   5% - 15%
    A. Electrophysiology and the Conduction System
        1. Propagation of electrical activity
        2. Excitation contraction coupling
    B. Mechanical Considerations and Events
        1. Frank Starling law (length-tension relationship)
        2. Force-velocity relationship
        3. Interval-strength relationship
        4. Valve opening and closure
    C. Phases of the Cardiac Cycle (Electro-mechanical Events)
        1. Passive filling phase (ventricular diastole)
        2. Atrial systole (p-wave on EKG; late diastole)
        3. Isovolumic contraction
        4. Ventricular ejection
        5. Isovolumic relaxation
    D. Left Ventricular Function; Indicators and Normal Values
        1. Stroke volume
        2. Ejection fraction

      3.   Cardiac output
  E. Pulmonary vs. Systemic Circulation; Differences and Similarities
  F. Intracardiac Pressures and Principles of Flow
      1.   Normal values
      2.   Changes during the cardiac cycle and relation to valve opening/closure
  G. Maneuvers Altering Cardiac Physiology
  H. Normal Heart Sound Generation and Timing
  I. Cardiovascular Circulation
      1.   Normal metabolic needs and their variations
      2.   Component parts of the circulation
      3.   Control mechanisms
      4.   Coronary circulation
      5.   Properties of blood: composition

V. Cardiac Evaluation Methods   5% - 15%
  A. Symptoms of Cardiac Diseases and Common Causes
  B. Physical Examination and Signs
      1.   General physical appearance and patient history
      2.   Correlation of auscultatory findings
         a.   Normal heart sounds
         b.   Abnormal heart sounds and common causes
         c.   Murmurs, timing, location, intensity, character, grading
  C. EKG
      1.   Basic principles and waveforms
      2.   Common abnormalities: basic pattern recognition
      3.   Exercise and pharmocologic stress testing: basic principles
  D. Phonocardiography: Basic Principles and Waveforms
  E. Cardiac Catheterization
      1.   Basic concepts of hemodynamic recordings
      2.   Determination of cardiac output
      3.   Oximetry
      4.   Coronary angiography
      5.   Evaluation and definition of gradients
      6.   Recognition of pressure wave forms in common disease states
  F. Other Diagnostic Modalities - Correlation to Echocardiography
      1.   Chest x-ray
      2.   Nuclear cardiology
      3.   Phonocardiography
  G. Relation of Cardiac Events as Recorded on ECG, Phonocardiogram, Presssure Tracings, etc.
  H. Correlation and Integration of Information Obtained with Echocardiography and Various Methods of Cardiac Evaluation
  I. Superimposed Respiratory Tracing
  J. Knowledge of CPR Techniques

VI. Principles of Cardiac Hemodynamics   5% - 15%
    A. Blood Flow Dynamics
        1. Factors affecting blood flow
        2. Laminar Flow: definition, characteristics, and types
        3. Disturbed Flow: definition, characteristics
        4. Relationships between pressure and velocity: Bernoulli principles and equations used
    B. Effects of Abnormal Pressures and Loading, Volume Concepts
        1. Heart failure and shock
        2. Valvular stenosis
        3. Valvular regurgitation
        4. Shunts
        5. Pulmonary disease
        6. Pericardial disease
        7. Cardiomyopathies

NORMAL HEART

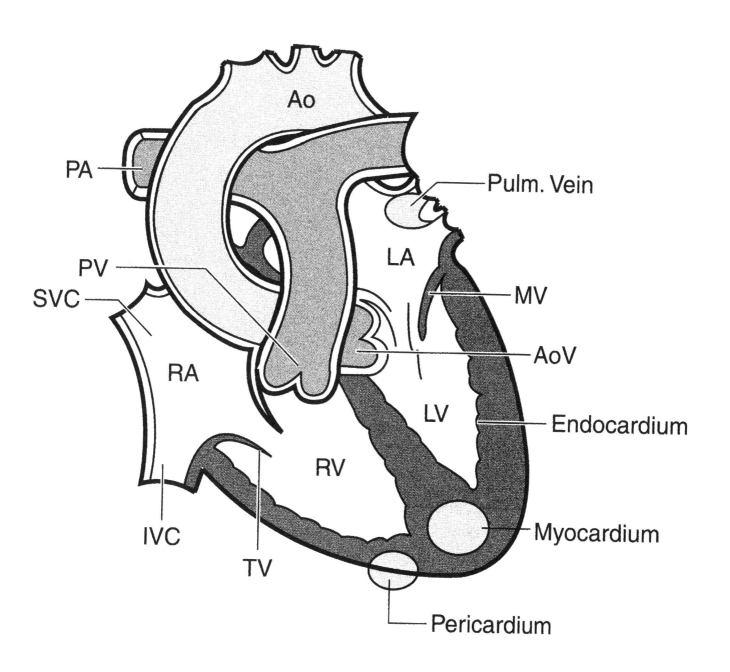

Ao

PA

Pulm. Vein

PV

LA

MV

SVC

AoV

RA

LV

Endocardium

IVC

RV

Myocardium

TV

Pericardium

CHAPTER 1 (UNIT ONE) - ANATOMY OF THE HEART

CHAPTER ONE
ANATOMY OF THE HEART

SECTION 1A
Chambers and Related Septa

The heart consists of four chambers: two receiving chambers (atria) and two pumping chambers (ventricles).

1. ATRIA (AURICLES)

The atria are the two upper receiving chambers which are separated by the interatrial septum.

Right Atrium (RA)

The right atrium receives deoxygenated blood from the superior vena cava (SVC), inferior vena cava (IVC), and the coronary sinus during ventricular systole and delivers blood into the right ventricle during ventricular diastole.

The RA consists of two chambers: the principal cavity which is composed, in part, of the posterior, smooth walled portion derived from the embryonic right atrium called the sinus venosus, and the atrial appendage.

The sulcus terminalis is a posterior external ridge that extends vertically from the superior vena cava to the inferior vena cava. The crista terminalis is an internal ridge that corresponds to the sulcus terminalis.

Along the RA free wall are a number of pectinate muscles that extend into the RA appendage.

The IVC is guarded by a vestigial valve at its entrance into the RA called the eustachian valve. Its fenestrated portion is referred to as the network of Chiari. The thebesian valve is a vestigial valve located at the entrance of the coronary sinus in the RA.

The right coronary and noncoronary aortic valve cusps of the aortic root contact the medial portion of the right atrium creating a slight bulge called the torus aorticus. The proximity of the aortic valve cusps and aortic root to the RA permits a sinus of Valsalva aneurysm to rupture into the right atrium.

Left Atrium (LA)

The left atrium receives oxygenated blood from the lungs via the four pulmonary veins during ventricular systole and delivers oxygenated blood to the left ventricle during ventricular diastole.

The LA consists of two chambers: the principal cavity and the left atrial appendage.

The left atrial free wall and left atrial appendage contain pectinate muscle.

The esophagus is located posterior to the left atrium.

The aortic root rests on the anterior wall of the left atrium.

Interatrial septum (IAS)

The interatrial septum divides the right atrium and left atrium into equal halves.

The central portion of the IAS is called the foramen ovale (open window) during fetal life and the fossa ovalis (closed window) after birth.

CHAPTER 1 (UNIT ONE) - ANATOMY OF THE HEART

The ridge that surrounds the fossa ovalis is called the limbus of the fossa ovalis and may be viewed anatomically from the right atrium.

In approximately 25% of adults, the foramen ovale never seals completely, and therefore patent foramen ovale is a relatively common echocardiographic finding.

2. VENTRICLES

The ventricles are the two lower pumping chambers that are separated by the interventricular septum. The inner wall of both ventricles are characterized by:

                        trabeculae carneae
                        papillary muscles
                        chordae tendineae

The trabeculae carneae are thick muscle bands located along the inner walls of the ventricles.

The papillary muscles of both ventricles are located below the atrioventricular valves. The papillary muscles which project from the trabeculae carneae may be single, or bifid, or occasionally there may be a row of muscles arising from the ventricular wall.

The chordae tendineae are strong fibrous cords that originate from the tips of the papillary muscles and attach to the atrioventricular valves.

Right Ventricle (RV)

The right ventricle receives deoxygenated blood from the right atrium during ventricular diastole and pumps this blood to the lungs via the main pulmonary artery during ventricular systole. It is thin walled as compared to the left ventricle because it pumps against a lower resistance. The right ventricle's pumping action has been likened to that of a fireplace bellows. The RV is the most anterior cardiac chamber and has a triangular shape exteriorly.

The RV is divided into three sections: inflow tract, apex and outflow tract.

The RV inflow tract includes the tricuspid valve annulus, three tricuspid valve leaflets, (anterior, posterior, septal), chordae tendineae, three papillary muscles and the RV myocardium. The names of the three RV papillary muscles are anterior, posterior and medial (conal).

The RV apex is heavily trabeculated, especially when compared to the left ventricle. The moderator band is a muscle band that lies near the RV apex. The moderator band stretches from the RV free wall to the interventricular septum and carries the conduction system's right bundle branch.

The RV outflow tract extends cephalad and leftward from the anterior-medial portion of the tricuspid valve annulus to the pulmonic valve annulus. It includes the smooth walled area beneath the pulmonic valve called the infundibulum. The crista supraventricularis is an anteriorly located muscle bundle that separates the RV inflow tract from the RV outflow tract. The conus arteriosus is a ridge or bump located externally where the right ventricular outflow tract meets the pulmonary artery.

Left Ventricle: (LV)

The thickest chamber, representing 75% of the heart's total mass, pumps oxygenated blood received from the left atrium during ventricular diastole into the ascending aorta during ventricular systole. The LV is thick walled because it pumps blood into the highly resistant systemic circulation.

The LV is divided into three sections: inflow tract, apex and outflow tract.

The LV inflow tract includes the mitral valve annulus, two mitral valve leaflets (anterior, posterior), chordae tendineae, two papillary muscles and the LV myocardium. The two LV papillary muscle sets are called anterolateral and posteromedial.

The LV normally forms the cardiac apex.

The LV outflow tract anatomically extends from the mitral valve annulus to the aortic valve annulus. Functionally the left ventricular outflow tract extends from the free edge of the anterior mitral valve leaflet to the aortic valve annulus.

The left ventricle is three times thicker than the right ventricle. The normal LV is considered to be a prolate ellipse.

Interventricular Septum (IVS)

The interventricular septum is a thick muscular wall that separates the RV and LV.

The majority of the IVS is muscular except for a small membranous portion located superiorly just beneath the right coronary aortic valve cusp. This thin portion of the IVS is called the membranous septum.

The muscular septum may be divided into three regions:

1. The inlet region, which lies inferior to the membranous septum between the two atrioventricular valves and comprises the superior-posterior one-third of the muscular septum.

2. The trabecular region is the largest region and extends from the membranous septum to the cardiac apex.

3. The infundibular or outlet region lies in the superior-anterior portion of the septum and lies superior to the trabecular septum and inferior to the great vessels.

Because normal left ventricular systolic and diastolic pressure is greater than right ventricular systolic and diastolic pressures, the IVS is concave to the LV and convex to the RV.

REVIEW PRACTICE - Section 1A

1. The heart has _____ chambers.

2. The heart has _____ receiving chambers and _____ pumping chambers.

3. The _____ are considered the heart's receiving chambers.

4. The _____ atrium is the receiving chamber of the right heart.

5. The right atrium receives deoxygenated blood from the _____ vena cava, _____ vena cava and the _____ sinus.

6. The right atrium fills during ventricular _____.

7. The _____ terminalis is a right atrial externally located ridge which runs from the superior vena cava to the inferior vena cava.

8. The _____ terminalis is a ridge located internally that corresponds to the sulcus terminalis.

9. The muscle bundles located along the free wall of the right atrium that extend into the right atrial appendage are called _____ muscles.

10. The inferior vena cava's entrance into the right atrium is guarded by a vestigial valve called the _____ valve.

11. The fenestrated portion of the eustachian valve is the _____ network.

12. The vestigial valve that guards the opening of the coronary sinus is the _____ valve.

13. The bulge created by the right coronary and noncoronary aortic valve cusps is called the _____ _____.

14. True or False: Due to the close proximity of the right coronary and noncoronary aortic valve cusps to the right atrium a ruptured sinus of Valsalva aneurysm may leak into the right atrium.

15. The _____ atrium is the receiving chamber of the left heart.

16. The left atrium receives oxygenated blood from the four _____ veins during ventricular systole.

17. The muscle bundles that striate the free wall of the left atrium and extend into the left atrial appendage are called _____ muscle.

18. True or False: The esophagus lies anterior to the left atrium.

19. The _____ septum divides the right atrium and left atrium into equal halves.

20. The open central portion of the interatrial septum during fetal life is called the _____ _____.

21. In the adult, the closed central portion of the interatrial septum is called the _____ _____.

22. Each ventricle contains _____ carneae, _____ muscles and _____ tendineae.

23. The _____ ventricle is the pumping chamber of the right heart.

CHAPTER 1 (UNIT ONE) - ANATOMY OF THE HEART

24. The right _____ accepts deoxygenated blood from the right atrium during ventricular diastole and pumps blood into the main pulmonary artery during ventricular systole.

25. The right ventricle is thick?/thin? walled.

26. True or False: The right ventricle is the most anterior cardiac chamber.

27. The right ventricle is made up of an _____ tract, apex and _____ tract.

28. True or False: The right ventricular inflow tract consists of the tricuspid valve annulus, tricuspid valve leaflets, chordae tendineae, papillary muscles and right ventricular myocardium.

29. The right ventricle contains three papillary muscle sets called _____, _____ and _____ or conal.

30. True or False: The right ventricular apex is heavily trabeculated.

31. The subpulmonic area of the right ventricle is called the _____.

32. The _____ _____ is an anteriorly located muscle bundle that separates the inflow and outflow tracts of the right ventricle.

33. The conus _____ is the external ridge located where the right ventricle meets the pulmonary artery.

34. The _____ band stretches from the free wall of the right ventricle to the interventricular septum.

35. The _____ ventricle is the pumping chamber of the left heart.

36. The _____ ventricle accepts oxygenated blood from the left atrium during ventricular diastole and pumps blood into the aorta during ventricular systole.

37. The left ventricle is thick?/thin? walled.

38. The left ventricle is made up of an _____ tract, apex and _____ tract.

39. True or False: The left ventricular inflow tract consists of the mitral annulus, mitral valve leaflets, chordae tendineae, papillary muscles and left ventricular myocardium.

40. The two papillary muscle sets of the left ventricle are the _____ and _____ papillary muscles.

41. True or False: The left ventricle normally forms the cardiac apex.

42. The shape of the normal left ventricle is assumed to be a prolate _____.

43. The _____ septum separates the right and left ventricles.

44. The two parts of the interventricular septum are the _____ septum and the _____ septum.

45. The muscular interventricular septum is divided into three regions called the _____, _____, and _____ regions.

46. The interventricular septum is _____ to the left ventricle and _____ to the right ventricle.

CHAPTER 1 (UNIT ONE) - ANATOMY OF THE HEART

BOARD REVIEW QUESTIONS - Section 1A

1. The heart has _____ chambers.
    a. 2
    b. 3
    c. 4
    d. 5

2. The right atrium receives deoxygenated blood from all of the following except:
    a. inferior vena cava
    b. superior vena cava
    c. pulmonary veins
    d. coronary sinus

3. The right atrium fills predominantly during:
    a. atrial systole
    b. ventricular diastole
    c. ventricular diastasis
    d. ventricular systole

4. The muscle bundles of the atria and appendages are called:
    a. trabeculae carneae
    b. pectinate muscle
    c. false tendons
    d. ectopic chordae

5. The vestigial valve that guards the opening of the inferior vena cava is the:
    a. thebesian
    b. tricuspid
    c. eustachian
    d. Chiari

6. The fenestrated portion of the eustachian valve is called the:
    a. limbus
    b. Chiari network
    c. membranous septum
    d. foramen ovale

7. The central opening of the interatrial septum during fetal circulation is called the:
    a. fossa ovalis
    b. eustachian
    c. foramen ovale
    d. Chiari network

CHAPTER 1 (UNIT ONE) - ANATOMY OF THE HEART

    c. crista terminalis
    d. infundibulum

9. The left atrium receives oxygenated blood from the pulmonary veins predominantly during ventricular:
    a. diastole
    b. diastasis
    c. systole
    d. repolarization

10. The closed central portion of the interatrial septum in the adult is called the:
    a. foramen ovale
    b. fossa ovalis
    c. thebesian valve
    d. ostium primum

11. The ventricles contain all of the following except:
    a. trabeculae carneae
    b. papillary muscles
    c. chordae tendineae
    d. pectinate muscles

12. All of the following are true statements concerning the right ventricle except:
    a. thick walled
    b. moderator band is located here
    c. contains three papillary muscle sets
    d. outflow portion called the infundibulum

13. The muscle bundle that separates the inflow tract from the outflow tract in the right ventricle is called the:
    a. crista terminalis
    b. crista supraventricularis
    c. sulcus terminalis
    d. torus aorticus

14. The names of the three papillary muscle groups of the right ventricle include all of the following except:
    a. lateral
    b. conal
    c. anterior
    d. posterior

15. All of the following are true statements concerning the left ventricle except:
    a. prolate ellipse in shape
    b. has two papillary muscle sets
    c. carries oxygenated blood
    d. high carbon dioxide content

16. The names of the two papillary muscle sets of the left ventricle are:
    a. anteromedial; posterior
    b. anterior; posterior
    c. anterolateral; posteromedial
    d. anterior; lateral

17. The portion of the interventricular septum located just beneath the aortic valve is the:
    a. muscular
    b. trabecular
    c. noncoronary
    d. membranous

18. All of the following are considered regions of the muscular interventricular septum except:
    a. trabecular
    b. inlet
    c. outlet
    d. primum

19. The interventricular septum normally bows towards the:
    a. right atrium
    b. right ventricle
    c. left atrium
    d. left ventricle

ANSWERS - Section 1A

Review practice answers

1. four
2. 2, 2
3. atria
4. right
5. superior, inferior, coronary
6. systole
7. sulcus
8. crista
9. pectinate
10. eustachian
11. Chiari
12. thebesian
13. torus aorticus
14. True
15. left
16. pulmonary
17. pectinate
18. False
19. interatrial
20. foramen ovale
21. fossa ovalis
22. trabeculae, papillary, chordae
23. right
24. ventricle
25. thin
26. True
27. inflow, outflow
28. True
29. anterior, posterior, medial
30. True
31. infundibulum
32. crista supraventricularis
33. arteriosus
34. moderator
35. left
36. left
37. thick
38. inflow, outflow
39. True
40. anterolateral, posteromedial
41. True

CHAPTER 1 (UNIT ONE) - ANATOMY OF THE HEART

42. ellipse
43. interventricular
44. membranous, muscular (trabecular)
45. inlet, trabecular, outlet
46. concave, convex

Board review answers

1. c
2. c
3. d
4. b
5. c
6. b
7. c
8. d
9. c
10. b
11. d
12. a
13. b
14. a
15. d
16. c
17. d
18. d
19. b

SECTION 1B
Valves and Related Apparatus

There are four cardiac valves: two atrioventricular valves and two semilunar valves. The cardiac valves regulate the flow of blood in the heart in one direction only while preventing backflow.

Atrioventricular Valves (AV)

The two AV valves are located between the atria and the ventricles. The AV valves are attached to the papillary muscles by chordae tendineae. The right heart AV valve is called the tricuspid valve and the left heart AV valve is called the mitral valve.

Tricuspid Valve

The tricuspid valve sits between the right atrium and right ventricle. It has 3 leaflets:
> anterior (largest)
> septal (medial)
> posterior

The tricuspid valve allows blood to flow from the RA to the RV during ventricular diastole and prevents the backflow of blood into the right atrium during ventricular systole.

The tricuspid valve apparatus includes the annulus, valve leaflets, chordae tendineae, three papillary muscles and the ventricular myocardium.

The posterior tricuspid valve leaflet has one to three sections called scallops.

Mitral Valve (bicuspid valve)

The mitral valve sits between the left atrium and left ventricle. It is composed of two leaflets and two commissures:
> anterior (largest)
> posterior
> lateral commissure
> medial commissure

The mitral valve apparatus includes the annulus, valve leaflets, chordae tendineae, two papillary muscles and the ventricular myocardium.

The posterior mitral valve leaflet has between one to three scallops called lateral, middle (largest) and medial.

Semilunar Valves

The semilunar valves are half-moon shaped valves that are situated at the mouth of the pulmonary artery and aorta.

Pulmonary Valve

The pulmonary valve sits between the right ventricle and main pulmonary artery and allows blood to flow from the RV to the main pulmonary artery during ventricular systole. During ventricular diastole, the 3 pulmonary valves prevent the backflow of blood. The names of the 3 pulmonary valve cusps are:

> right
> left (posterior)
> anterior

The point at which two adjacent cusps come together is called a commissure. At the tip of each pulmonic valve cusp is a small nodule called the nodule of Atlantii. In the mid-portion of each cusp is a slight indentation called the lunula. Behind each pulmonic valve cusp is a pouchlike dilatation called a sinus.

Aortic Valve

The aortic valve consists of 3 semilunar valve cusps which sit at the mouth of the aorta. The aortic valve allows blood to flow from the left ventricle to the aorta during ventricular systole and prevents the backflow of blood into the left ventricle during ventricular diastole. The names of the three aortic valve cusps are:

> right coronary
> left coronary
> noncoronary

Each aortic valve cusp has a commissure, a lunula, a nodule of Arantii and a sinus of Valsalva. Portions of the left coronary and noncoronary aortic valve cusps are continuous with the anterior mitral valve leaflet. The most common congenital heart defect in the adult population is the bicuspid aortic valve.

REVIEW PRACTICE - Section 1B

1. True or False: The cardiac valves regulate the flow of blood in the heart.

2. The _____ valves are located between the atria and the ventricles.

3. The atrioventricular valves are connected to the papillary muscles via the _____ _____.

4. The tricuspid valve has _____ leaflets.

5. The names of the three tricuspid valve leaflets are: _____, _____ and _____.

6. The _____ tricuspid valve leaflet is the largest of the three leaflets.

7. True or False: The posterior tricuspid valve leaflet may have one to three scallops.

8. True or False: The tricuspid valve is the atrioventricular valve that normally allows blood to flow from the right atrium to the right ventricle during ventricular systole.

9. True or False: The tricuspid valve prevents the backflow of blood from the right ventricle to the right atrium during ventricular systole.

10. The _____ valve is the atrioventricular valve that sits between the left atrium and left ventricle.

11. The mitral valve has _____ leaflets and _____ commissures.

12. The names of the two mitral valve leaflets are the _____ mitral valve leaflet and the _____ mitral valve leaflet.

13. The name of the two mitral commissures are the _____ commissure and the _____ commissure.

14. True or False: The posterior mitral valve leaflet may have one to three scallops.

15. The names of the three posterior mitral valve scallops are _____, _____ and _____.

16. The _____ scallop of the posterior mitral valve leaflet is the largest scallop.

17. True or False: The mitral valve allows blood to flow from the left atrium to the left ventricle during ventricular diastole.

18. True or False: The mitral valve prevents the backflow of blood from the left ventricle to the left atrium during ventricular systole.

19. The _____ valves are the half moon shaped valves that sit between the ventricles and the great vessels.

20. The _____ valve sits between the right ventricle and the main pulmonary artery.

21. True or False: The pulmonary valve allows blood to flow from the right ventricle to the main pulmonary artery during ventricular systole.

22. True or False: The pulmonary valve prevents the backflow of blood from the main pulmonary artery to the right ventricle during ventricular diastole.

23. The names of the three pulmonary valve cusps are the _____, _____ and _____.

24. True or False: The posterior pulmonary valve cusp is also called the left cusp.

25. True or False: All of the following are components of the pulmonary valve cusps: commissures, nodules of Atlantii, lunula and sinuses.

26. True or False: The aortic valve cusps allow blood to flow from the left ventricle to the aorta during ventricular systole.

27. True or False: The aortic valve prevents the backflow of blood from the aorta to the left ventricle during ventricular diastole.

28. The names of the three aortic valve cusps are the _____, _____ and _____- coronary cusps.

29. True or False: All of the following are components of the aortic valve cusps: commissures, nodules of Arantii, lunula and the sinuses of Valsalva.

30. The _____ coronary and _____coronary aortic valve cusps are contiguous with the anterior mitral valve leaflet.

31. The most common adult congenital heart lesion is the _____ aortic valve.

BOARD REVIEW QUESTIONS - Section 1B

1. The valves that regulate blood flow between the atria and ventricles during ventricular systole and diastole are called the:
   a. atrioventricular
   b. semilunar
   c. vestigial
   d. rudimentary

2. All of the following are components of the atrioventricular valves except:
   a. papillary muscles
   b. chordae tendineae
   c. valve leaflets
   d. chordal web

3. The names of the three tricuspid valve leaflets include all of the following except:
   a. anterior
   b. medial
   c. posterior
   d. left

4. The largest of the three tricuspid valve leaflets is the:
   a. anterior
   b. medial
   c. septal
   d. posterior

5. The mitral valve includes all of the following except:
   a. anterior leaflet
   b. medial commissure
   c. lateral commissure
   d. medial leaflet

6. The names of the three posterior mitral valve leaflet scallops include all of the following except:
   a. anterior
   b. middle
   c. medial
   d. lateral

7. The name of the cardiac valve that regulates blood flow from the ventricles to the great vessels during ventricular systole and diastole is:
   a. atrioventricular
   b. semilunar
   c. vestigial
   d. rudimentary

CHAPTER 1 (UNIT ONE) - ANATOMY OF THE HEART

8. All of the following are considered components of the semilunar valve cusps except:
    a. lunula
    b. commissures
    c. nodules (Atlantii, Arantii)
    d. chordae

9. The names of the three pulmonary valve cusps include all of the following except:
    a. anterior
    b. right
    c. posterior
    d. medial

10. The names of the three aortic valve cusps include all of the following except:
    a. anterior
    b. right
    c. left
    d. non-coronary

CHAPTER 1 (UNIT ONE) - ANATOMY OF THE HEART

ANSWERS - Section 1B

Review practice answers

1.   True
2.   atrioventricular
3.   chordae tendineae
4.   three
5.   anterior, medial (septal), posterior
6.   anterior
7.   True
8.   False
9.   True
10. mitral
11   two, two
12. anterior, posterior
13. medial, lateral
14. True
15. lateral, middle, medial
16. middle
17. True
18. True
19. semilunar
20. pulmonary
21. True
22. True
23. anterior, posterior (left), right
24. True
25. True
26. True
27. True
28. right, left, non
29   True
30. left, non
31. bicuspid

Board review answers

1.   a   8.   d
2.   d   9.   d
3.   d   10. a
4.   a
5.   d
6.   a
7.   b

CHAPTER 1 (UNIT ONE) - ANATOMY OF THE HEART

SECTION 1C
Arterial - Venous system

1. ARTERIES

The arteries are a network of thick-walled vessels that carry oxygenated blood throughout the body.

Aorta

The aorta carries oxygenated blood from the left ventricle to the rest of the body. The aorta is divided into the following sections:

>aortic annulus
>aortic root
>sinotubular junction
>ascending aorta
>aortic arch (transverse aorta)
>descending thoracic aorta
>abdominal aorta

The aortic arch gives off three vessels:

>brachiocephalic (innominate)
>left common carotid
>left subclavian

The aortic isthmus is a small section of the aorta which extends from the left subclavian artery to the insertion of the ligamentum arteriosum (ductus arteriosus).

Coronary arteries

The coronary arteries supply oxygenated blood to the heart muscle. The two coronary arteries originate from the right and left sinuses of Valsalva respectively.

Right coronary artery

The right coronary artery originates from the right sinus of Valsalva, proceeds anteriorly in the right atrioventricular coronary sulcus, and then winds around the RA and RV posteriorly. In 67% of humans, the posterior descending artery, which lies in the posterior interventricular sulcus, is a branch of the right coronary artery that supplies oxygenated blood to the inferior surface of the heart.

The right coronary artery also supplies oxygenated blood to the right atrium, sinoatrial and atrioventricular nodes and the right ventricle.

Left coronary artery

The left main coronary artery originates from the left sinus of Valsalva, and after traveling about 1 centimeter bifurcates into the left anterior descending (LAD) and the left circumflex. The LAD lies in the anterior interventricular sulcus and divides the RV and LV anteriorly. The LAD supplies oxygenated blood to the anterior interventricular septum via branches called septal perforators, the anterior wall of the left ventricle through branches called diagonals and the cardiac apex. The left circumflex lies in the left atrioventricular coronary sulcus and winds around the left side of the heart dividing the LA and LV anteriorly and posteriorly.

The circumflex mainly supplies oxygenated blood to the lateral walls of the left ventricle via branches called marginals. The circumflex also supplies the left atrium with oxygenated blood.

Pulmonary Artery

The pulmonary artery connects the right ventricle to the lungs.

The main pulmonary artery originates at the summit of the right ventricle and bifurcates into the left pulmonary artery and right pulmonary artery.

The pulmonary artery is the only artery in the body to carry deoxygenated blood.

2. VEINS

Veins are thin-walled vessels that are smaller than arteries, and which carry deoxygenated blood to the heart.

Superior Vena Cava (SVC)

The superior vena cava returns deoxygenated blood from the head and arms to the heart via the right atrium.

Inferior Vena Cava (IVC)

The inferior vena cava returns deoxygenated blood from below the heart (trunk and legs) to the right atrium.

The valve that guards the opening of the IVC is the eustachian valve with the fenestrated portion called the network of Chiari.

Coronary sinus

The coronary sinus collects deoxygenated blood from the coronary arteries and returns the heart's blood to the right atrium.

The coronary sinus has three tributaries:

Great cardiac vein, which drains the left anterior descending and circumflex coronary arteries.

Middle cardiac vein, which drains the posterior descending coronary artery

Small cardiac vein, which drains the right coronary artery.

The thebesian, arterioluminal, and arteriosinusoidal are small cardiac veins that empty a small portion of the coronary venous circulation directly into the cardiac chambers.

Pulmonary veins

The pulmonary veins are four vessels that deliver oxygenated blood to the left atrium. They are referred to as the right upper, right lower, left upper and left lower. They are the only veins in the body that carry oxygenated blood. There are three components to pulmonary venous flow: systolic (S wave), early ventricular diastole (D wave), and the atrial reversal (AR wave) which occurs during atrial systole.

REVIEW PRACTICE - Section 1C

1. The _____ are a network of thick walled vessels that carry oxygenated blood throughout the body.

2. Check the following if considered a part of the aorta:

    _____aortic annulus

    _____aortic root

    _____ascending aorta

    _____aortic arch

    _____descending thoracic aorta

    _____abdominal aorta

3. The aortic arch gives of three vessels. They are: _____, left common _____, left _____ arteries.

4. The aortic _____ is a small section of the aorta which is located between the left subclavian artery and the insertion of the ligamentum arteriosum.

5. The two coronary arteries originate from the sinuses of _____.

6. The _____ coronary artery provides oxygenated blood to the right atrium, sinoatrial node, atrioventricular node and the right ventricle.

7. In 67% of humans, the right coronary artery sends the _____ descending artery which provides oxygenated blood to the inferior interventricular septum and the inferior walls of the right and left ventricles.

8. The left coronary artery bifurcates into the left _____ descending artery and the left _____ artery.

9. True or False: The left anterior descending coronary artery supplies oxygenated blood to the anterior interventricular septum via septal perforators, anterior wall of the left ventricle via the diagonal branches and the cardiac apex.

10. True or False: The left circumflex coronary artery provides oxygenated blood to the left atrium and, via the oblique marginal branches, the lateral walls of the left ventricle.

11. The _____ artery connects the right ventricle to the lungs.

12. The main pulmonary artery bifurcates into the _____ and _____ pulmonary artery branches.

13. _____ are thinner walled than arteries and carry deoxygenated blood to the heart.

14. The _____ vena cava returns deoxygenated blood to the heart from the upper part of the body.

15. The _____ vena cava returns deoxygenated blood to the heart from the lower part of the body.

16. The _____ sinus returns deoxygenated blood to the heart from the coronary arteries.

17. The coronary sinus receives deoxygenated blood from three tributaries. They are the _____ cardiac vein, _____ cardiac vein, and _____ cardiac vein.

18. The _____ veins deliver oxygenated blood to the left atrium.

19. The three components to pulmonary venous flow are the _____ wave, _____ wave and the _____ wave.

20. Normally, the pulmonary vein S wave?/D wave?/AR wave? is the predominant wave.

BOARD REVIEW QUESTIONS - Section 1C

1. Which of the following carry oxygenated blood throughout the body?
    a. arteries
    b. veins
    c. venules
    d. vasa vasorum

2. All of the following are considered sections of the aorta except:
    a. annulus
    b. root
    c. right/left branches
    d. arch

3. All of the following arteries originate from the aortic arch except:
    a. left subclavian
    b. right subclavian
    c. left common carotid
    d. brachiocephalic

4. The small section of the aorta located between the left subclavian artery and the insertion of the ligamentum arteriosum is the aortic:
    a. arch
    b. annulus
    c. isthmus
    d. coarctation

5. The coronary arteries originate from the sinuses of:
    a. Bernheim
    b. Carvallo
    c. Bernoulli
    d. Valsalva

6. Which coronary artery provides oxygenated blood to the inferior interventricular septum, and inferior walls of the left and right ventricles?
    a. left main
    b. posterior descending
    c. circumflex
    d. left anterior descending

7. In the majority of human hearts, the posterior descending artery is a branch of which coronary artery?
    a. right
    b. left
    c. circumflex
    d. anterior descending

8. The right coronary artery provides oxygenated blood to all of the following except the:
    a. right atrium
    b. left atrium
    c. sinoatrial node
    d. right ventricle

9. The two branches of the left coronary artery are the:
    a. anterolateral, posteromedial
    b. diagonal, posterior descending
    c. anterior descending, circumflex
    d. circumflex, acute marginal

10. The left anterior descending coronary artery provides oxygenated blood to all of the following except the:
    a. anterior interventricular septum
    b. inferior interventricular septum
    c. anterior wall of the left ventricle
    d. cardiac apex

11. The circumflex coronary artery provides oxygenated blood to all of the following except the:
    a. anterior wall of the left ventricle
    b. anterolateral wall of the left ventricle
    c. left atrium
    d. lateral wall of the left ventricle

12. Which of the following vessels connect the right ventricle to the lungs?
    a. main pulmonary
    b. aorta
    c. vena cava
    d. pulmonary veins

13. All of the following veins carry deoxygenated blood except the:
    a. superior vena cava
    b. inferior vena cava
    c. coronary sinus
    d. pulmonary veins

CHAPTER 1 (UNIT ONE) - ANATOMY OF THE HEART

14. The coronary sinus receives deoxygenated blood from all of the following veins except:
    a. great cardiac
    b. middle cardiac
    c. small cardiac
    d. posterior cardiac

15. Pulmonary venous flow normally occurs predominantly during:
    a. ventricular diastole
    b. atrial systole
    c. ventricular systole
    d. cannot be predicted

ANSWERS - Section 1C

Review practice answers

1. arteries
2. all
3. innominate (brachiocephalic), carotid, subclavian
4. isthmus
5. Valsalva
6. right
7. posterior
8. anterior, circumflex
9. True
10. True
11. pulmonary
12. right, left
13. veins
14. superior
15. inferior
16. coronary
17. great, middle, small
18. pulmonary
19. S, D, AR
20. S wave

Board review answers

1. a.
2. c
3. b
4. c
5. d
6. b
7. a
8. b
9. c
10. b
11. a
12. a
13. d
14. d
15. c

CHAPTER 1 (UNIT ONE) - ANATOMY OF THE HEART

Section 1D
Conduction System

The cardiac conduction system consists of the following components:

Sino-atrial Node (SA)

The sino-atrial node is the pacemaker of the heart. It fires electrical impulses 60-100 times per minute. The SA node is an oval shaped group of specialized cells located at the roof of the RA near the entrance of the superior vena cava. The SA node is oxygenated usually by the right coronary artery.

Internodal pathways

The internodal pathways carry the electrical impulse to both atria. The most developed is Bachmann's bundle which carries the impulse from the SA node to the left atrium.

Atrioventricular Node (AV)

Located at the floor of the RA near the septal leaflet of the tricuspid valve, the AV node delays the impulse 1/10th of a second in order for the atria to completely deliver blood to the ventricles. The AV node is oxygenated by the right coronary artery.

Bundle of His (AV Bundle)

This thin bundle is a continuation of the AV node and carries the electrical impulse to the bundle branches.

Right/Left Bundle Branches

The bundle branches run along the right and left side of the interventricular septum and carry the electrical impulse to the ventricles. The bundle branches blood supply comes from both the right and left coronary arteries.

Purkinje Fibers

The fiber network that delivers the electrical impulse to the ventricular heart wall (endocardium) causing depolarization of the ventricles. Depolarization occurs from inside to out (endocardium to epicardium) and from cardiac apex to the base of the heart.

REVIEW PRACTICE - Section 1D

1. The pacemaker of the heart is the _____ atrial node.

2. The sinoatrial node normally fires _____-_____ times per minute.

3. The _____ pathways deliver the electrical impulse from the SA node to the atria.

4. The most developed internodal pathway is _____ bundle.

5. The _____ node delays the electrical impulse in order for the atria to completely deliver blood to the ventricles.

6. The bundle of _____ carries the electrical impulse to the bundle branches.

7. The _____ bundle branch carries the electrical impulse to the right ventricle.

8. The _____ bundle branch carries the electrical impulse to the left ventricle.

9. The _____ fibers deliver the electrical impulse to the ventricular endocardium which causes depolarization of the ventricles.

10. The SA node and the AV node receive oxygenated blood from the _____ coronary artery.

11. True or False: The left ventricle normally depolarizes slightly before the right ventricle.

BOARD REVIEW QUESTIONS - Section 1D

1. The pacemaker of the heart is the:
    a. sinoatrial node
    b. internodal pathways
    c. atrioventricular node
    d. bundle of His

2. Which of the following carries the electrical impulse from the sinoatrial node to the atria?
    a. internodal pathways
    b. atrioventricular node
    c. His bundle
    d. Purkinje fibers

3. The most developed internodal pathway that carries the electrical impulse to the left atrium is:
    a. Thorel
    b. Bachmann's
    c. Wenckebach
    d. His

4. Which of the following delays the electrical impulse to allow the atria to deliver blood to the ventricles?
    a. sinoatrial node
    b. internodal pathways
    c. atrioventricular node
    d. Purkinje fibers

5. Which of the following carries the electrical impulse from the atria to the ventricles?
    a. sinoatrial node
    b. internodal pathways
    c. atrioventricular node
    d. His bundle

6. Which of the following carries the electrical impulse to the ventricles?
    a. sinoatrial node
    b. internodal pathways
    c. His bundle
    d. bundle branches

7. Which of the following delivers the electrical impulse to the ventricles causing ventricular depolarization?
    a. sinoatrial node
    b. internodal pathways
    c. bundle branches
    d. Purkinje fibers

ANSWERS - Section 1D

Review practice answers

1. sino
2. 60, 100
3. internodal
4. Bachmann's
5. atrioventricular (AV)
6. His
7. right
8. left
9. Purkinje
10. right
11. True

Board review answers

1. a
2. a
3. b
4. c
5. d
6. d
7. d

Section 1E
Layers of the Heart

The heart is made up of 3 distinct layers, plus the pericardium, the protective sac that surrounds the heart.

Epicardium

The epicardium is the thin outer layer directly adherent to the heart. It may also be referred to as the visceral pericardium.

Myocardium

The myocardium is the thick, middle muscular layer of the heart. Adipose tissue is fitted between the epicardium and myocardium.

Endocardium

The endocardium is the inner layer that is composed of endothelial cells, which line the heart's cavities and valves.

Pericardium

The pericardium is the protective sac that surrounds the heart. It is composed of the fibrous (parietal) pericardium, which is a tough, fibrous membrane that surrounds the heart and great vessels, and a thin inner membrane which lines the fibrous pericardium, called the parietal serous pericardium.

The pericardial cavity is the space located between the visceral and parietal layers. It normally contains up to 50 cc of fluid. The pressure in the pericardial cavity is normally negative, although it may increase during ventricular filling.

The pericardium creates free spaces or sinuses as it wraps around the base of the heart. These sinuses are called the:

Oblique sinus: A free space that is created by the pericardium wrapping around the pulmonary veins posteriorly.

Transverse sinus: A free space created by the pericardium wrapping around the base of the great vessels.

WALLS OF THE HEART

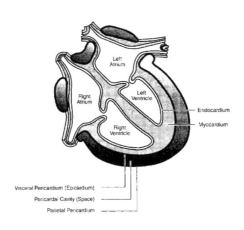

REVIEW PRACTICE - Section 1E

1. The three layers of the heart are the: _____, _____ and _____.

2. The outer layer of the heart is called the _____ or the _____ pericardium.

3. The middle muscular layer of the heart wall is the _____.

4. The inner lining of the heart is the _____.

5. True or False: Adipose tissue is located between the epicardium and myocardium.

6. The fibrous (parietal) _____ is the protective sac that covers the heart.

7. True or False: The parietal serous pericardium lines the fibrous pericardium.

8. The pericardial _____ is located between the visceral and parietal serous layers and normally contains up to 50 cc of fluid.

9. True or False: Normally the intrapericardial pressure is predominantly positive.

10. The _____ sinus is a free space located behind the left atrium created by the pericardial-pulmonary vein interface.

11. The _____ sinus is a free space located between the great vessels caused by the pericardial great vessel interface.

BOARD REVIEW QUESTIONS - Section 1E

1. The three layers of the heart include all of the following except:
    a. epicardium
    b. myocardium
    c. endocardium
    d. pericardium

2. The outer layer of the heart is the:
    a. epicardium
    b. myocardium
    c. endocardium
    d. pericardium

3. The middle, muscular layer of the heart is the:
    a. epicardium
    b. myocardium
    c. endocardium
    d. pericardium

4. The inner layer of the heart which also lines the cardiac valves is the:
    a. epicardium
    b. myocardium
    c. endocardium
    d. pericardium

5. Adipose tissue around the heart is located between the:
    a. visceral pericardium and fibrous pericardium
    b. epicardium and myocardium
    c. myocardium and endocardium
    d. endocardium and epicardium

6. The sac that surrounds the heart is the:
    a. parietal pericardium
    b. visceral pericardium
    c. epicardium
    d. endocardium

7. The thin membrane that lines the fibrous pericardium is called the:
    a. parietal serous
    b. epicardium
    c. myocardium
    d. endocardium

CHAPTER 1 (UNIT ONE) - ANATOMY OF THE HEART

8. The pericardial space is located between the:
    a. epicardium and myocardium
    b. endocardium and epicardium
    c. parietal serous pericardium and epicardium
    d. fibrous pericardium and endocardium

9. The posterior free space created by the pericardial-pulmonary vein interface is the:
    a. coronary sinus
    b. oblique sinus
    c. transverse sinus
    d. sinus of Valsalva

10. The free space created at the base of the heart by the pericardial-great vessel interface is the:
    a. coronary sinus
    b. oblique sinus
    c. transverse sinus
    d. sinus of Valsalva

CHAPTER 1 (UNIT ONE) - ANATOMY OF THE HEART

ANSWERS - Section 1E

Review practice answers

1. epicardium (visceral pericardium), myocardium, endocardium
2. epicardium, visceral
3. myocardium
4. endocardium
5. True
6. pericardium
7. True
8. space
9. False
10. oblique
11. transverse

Board review answers

1. d
2. a
3. b
4. c
5. b
6. a
7. a
8. c
9. b
10. c

Section 1F
Relational Anatomy

The heart lies underneath the sternum in the mediastinal cavity with one-third of the heart lying to the right of midline and two-thirds to the left of midline. Behind the heart is a small space called the retrocardiac space.

The apex of the heart is the blunt, rounded bottom of the heart which is located anteriorly and to the left. The base of the heart is located under the second rib, is the widest portion of the heart, and is located posteriorly and to the right.

The crux of the heart is the area where all four chambers meet posteriorly. Internally the crux of the heart refers to where the interatrial septum and interventricular septum meet.

The heart border where the left ventricle meets the lung is called the oblique margin. The heart border where the right ventricle meets the diaphragm is called the acute margin.

The heart moves downward (base to apex), twists counterclockwise and moves anteriorly during ventricular systole.

The average normal adult heart weighs 325 grams for men and 275 grams for women.

The heart's apparent shape may be altered by thoracic cage abnormalities (i.e. pectus excavatum).

The anterior interventricular sulcus divides the right and left ventricle anteriorly. The left anterior descending coronary artery is embedded in this sulcus.

The posterior interventricular sulcus divides the right and left ventricles posteriorly. The posterior descending coronary artery is embedded in this sulcus.

The right atrioventricular coronary sulcus separates the right atrium and right ventricle anteriorly and posteriorly. The right coronary artery is embedded in this sulcus.

The left atrioventricular coronary sulcus separates the left atrium and left ventricle anteriorly and posteriorly. The left circumflex coronary artery is embedded in this sulcus.

The pulmonary artery and valve lies anterior, superior and to the left of the aorta and aortic valve.

Compared to the mitral valve, the tricuspid valve is inserted closer to the cardiac apex.

REVIEW PRACTICE - Section 1F

1. True or False: The heart lies underneath the sternum in the mediastinum.

2. The _____ of the heart is the blunt, rounded bottom of the heart which is located anteriorly and to the left.

3. The _____ of the heart is widest part of the heart.

4. The pulmonary artery in comparison to the aorta lies anteriorly?/posteriorly?, superiorly?/inferiorly? and to the left?/right?

5. The tricuspid valve?/mitral valve? is inserted closer to the cardiac apex.

6. The left margin of the heart is called the _____ margin.

7. Where the diaphragm meets the right ventricle is called the _____ margin.

8. During ventricular systole, the heart moves _____, twists _____ and moves _____.

9. The left anterior descending coronary artery is embedded in the anterior _____ sulcus.

10. The posterior descending coronary artery is embedded in the posterior _____ sulcus.

11. The left circumflex coronary artery is embedded in the left _____ coronary sulcus.

12. The right coronary artery is embedded in the right _____ coronary sulcus.

13. Externally where all four cardiac chambers meet posteriorly is called the cardiac _____.

14. Internally where the interatrial septum meets the interventricular septum is called the cardiac _____.

BOARD REVIEW QUESTIONS- Section 1F

1. The heart lies beneath the:
    a. diaphragm
    b. sternum
    c. liver
    d. abdominal cavity

2. The tip of the heart is called the:
    a. base
    b. apex
    c. pericardium
    d. isthmus

3. The widest portion of the heart located beneath the second rib is the:
    a. base
    b. apex
    c. pericardium
    d. isthmus

4. In relation to the aorta, the pulmonary artery lies:
    a. anteriorly, rightward
    b. posteriorly; rightward
    c. anteriorly; leftward
    d. laterally; posteriorly

5. Which cardiac valve lies closest to the cardiac apex?
    a. mitral
    b. aortic
    c. pulmonic
    d. tricuspid

6. The circumflex coronary artery feeds the left border of the heart called the:
    a. acute margin
    b. oblique margin
    c. transverse sinus
    d. coronary sinus

7. All of the following describe the heart's motion during ventricular systole except:
    a. anteriorly
    b. laterally
    c. counterclockwise
    d. downward

CHAPTER 1 (UNIT ONE) - ANATOMY OF THE HEART

8. Where the interatrial septum meets the interventricular septum internally is called the cardiac:

    a. apex

    b. base

    c. truncus

    d. crux

ANSWERS - Section 1F

Review practice answers

1. True
2. apex
3. base
4. anteriorly, superiorly, left
5. tricuspid valve
6. oblique
7. acute
8. downward, counterclockwise, anteriorly
9. interventricular
10. interventricular
11. atrioventricular
12. atrioventricular
13. crux
14. crux

Board review answers

1. b
2. b
3. a
4. c
5. d
6. b
7. b
8. d

CHAPTER 1 (UNIT ONE) - ANATOMY OF THE HEART

CHAPTER TWO
BASIC EMBRYOLOGY

SECTION A.   Primitive Heart Tube

SECTION B.   Comparison of Fetal and Postnatal Circulation

SECTION 2A
Primitive Heart Tube

1. FORMATION FROM PRIMITIVE VASCULAR TUBE

The heart tube appears by week three and begins to beat by day 23. The heart is completely formed by week seven, and is the first organ to fully develop in the fetus.

The heart tube loops anteriorly and rightward creating the bulboventricular loop. The opening between the primitive ventricle (left ventricle) and the bulbus cordis (right ventricle) is called the bulboventricular foramen.

The regions of the heart tube below are presented as blood flows through the fetal heart tube (caudad to cephalad):

Sinus venosus
Primitive atria
Atrioventricular (AV) canal
Primitive ventricle
Bulbus cordis
Truncus arteriosus
Aortic sac and arches

Sinus Venosus

The sinus venosus consists of two horns, right and left, which eventually will contribute to the formation of the superior vena cava, inferior vena cava, coronary sinus and the posterior wall of the atria. The distal portion of the left horn usually dissipates, but if it persists it becomes a persistent left superior vena cava entering the coronary sinus or left atrium.

Primitive Atria

The primitive atria is divided equally by the interatrial septum, which is composed of the septum primum, septum secundum and the foramen ovale. The septum primum grows downward and anteriorly from the roof of the primitive atria, fuses with the endocardial cushions and develops a central perforation and opening that becomes the foramen ovale. The septum secundum originates from the atrial wall to the right of the septum primum and grows downward and posteriorly. The overresorption of the septum primum may result in a secundum atrial septal defect.

Atrioventricular (AV) Canal

The atrioventricular canal is a large communication between the primitive atria and primitive ventricle. The endocardial cushions will divide the AV canal into the two atrioventricular orifices as well as contribute to the closure of the ostium primum (inferior) portion of the atrial septum and membranous section of the interventricular septum. The endocardial cushions are also responsible for the formation of the anterior mitral valve leaflet and tricuspid valve septal leaflet. Complete absence of the endocardial cushions will result in a complete atrioventricular septal defect which is a common finding in Down's syndrome. Forty percent of Down's patients have atrioventricular septal defect.

Primitive Ventricle

The primitive ventricle is normally a morphologic left ventricle which shifts leftward during cardiac development and is eventually divided by the interventricular septum. Nearly 80% of univentricular hearts consist predominantly of a morphologic left ventricle.

Bulbus Cordis

The bulbus cordis is divided into three sections: primitive right ventricle, ventricular outflow tracts (conus cordis) and the truncus arteriosus. Cono-truncal abnormalities include truncus arteriosus and tetralogy of Fallot.

The truncus arteriosus contributes to the formation of the aorta and pulmonary artery trunks. Failure of the truncus to divide may result in persistent truncus arteriosus.

2. SINUS VENOSUS

The sinus venosus consists of a central portion called the transverse sinus, the right sinus horn and the left sinus horn. The left and right sinus horns receive three pairs of veins: the vitelline veins, the umbilical veins and the common cardinal veins. The proximal left sinus horn contributes to the formation of the coronary sinus while the distal left horn and veins normally obliterate.The right sinus horn contributes to the formation of the posterior wall of the right atrium called the sinus venarum, eustachian valve and thebesian valve. Persistence of the distal left sinus horn and left common cardinal vein results in a persistent left superior vena cava connected to the coronary sinus or left atrium.

3. CARDIAC LOOP

At approximately three weeks, the growing bulboventricular tube loops anterior and rightward creating the bulboventricular loop. The looping of the heart tube influences the spiral disposition of the truncoconal septum, displaces the atrioventricular canal laterally and to the left while the primitive ventricle shifts to the left side of the pericardial cavity. If the cardiac tube loops anterior and leftward instead of anterior and rightward, ventricular inversion (l-transposition, corrected transposition) will result.

4. AORTIC ARCHES

The aortic sac gives rise to six paired arches with three arches normally persisting. The third arch becomes the internal carotid artery, the fourth contributes to the formation of the aortic arch and the sixth will develop into the right and left pulmonary arteries and the ductus arteriosus. The aortic sac itself contributes to the formation of the ascending aorta. Persistence of the fourth arch may lead to a double aortic arch.

5. SEPTATION

Septation of the fetal heart is accomplished by the formation of seven septa. Three of the seven are formed passively: the atrial septum secundum, the muscular section of the interventricular septum and the aorticopulmonary septum. Three septa are formed actively: the atrioventricular canal septum, the conal septum and the truncal septum. The atrial septum primum begins as a passively formed septa but its closure is formed actively from the endocardial cushions.

6. VALVE FORMATION

The atrioventricular valves are derived primarily from the internal layer of the muscular ventricular wall. The arterial valves originate from small tubercles located at the proximal portion of aorta and pulmonary artery respectively.

REVIEW PRACTICE - Section 2A

1. The heart tube appears by week _____.

2. The heart is completely formed by week _____.

3. The heart tube loops _____ and _____ward.

4. The junction between the primitive ventricle and the bulbus cordis is called the _____ loop or tube.

5. The opening between the primitive ventricle and the bulbus cordis is the _____ foramen.

6. The seven distinct sections of the heart tube are: _____, _____, _____, _____, _____, _____, and _____ _____.

7. The _____ _____ contributes to the formation of the superior vena cava, inferior cava, coronary sinus and posterior wall of the right atrium and left atrium.

8. True or False: A persistent left superior vena cava is a result of the left horn of the sinus venosus remaining.

9. The _____ _____ will eventually be divided into the left atrium and right atrium.

10. The primitive atria is divided by the septum _____ and septum _____.

11. The central portion of the interatrial septum is called the _____ _____ in the fetal heart.

12. True or False: Overresoption of the septum primum may result in an ostium secundum atrial septal defect.

13. The _____ canal is a large communication between the primitive atria and primitive ventricle.

14. The _____ cushions divide the AV canal into the right and left atrioventricular orifices, contributes to the closure of the ostium primum and membranous septum and forms the anterior mitral valve and septal tricuspid valve leaflets.

15. True or False: Failure of the endocardial cushions may result in a complete atrioventricular canal septal defect.

16. The _____ _____ develops into the left ventricle.

17. True or False: 80% of univentricular hearts are morphologic left ventricles.

18. The _____ _____ contributes to the formation of the right ventricle, ventricular outflow tracts and truncus arteriosus.

19. The _____ _____ contributes to the formation of the aorta and pulmonary artery roots.

20. True or False: Failure of the truncus arteriosus to divide may result in persistent truncus arteriosus.

21. There are _____ paired aortic arches.

22. The _____ aortic arch contributes to the formation of the internal carotid artery.

23. The _____ aortic arch contributes to the formation of the aortic arch.

24. The _____ aortic arch contributes to the formation of the right and left pulmonary arteries and the ductus arteriosus.

25. The aortic _____ contributes to the formation of the ascending aorta.

26. True or False: Normally, the cardiac tube loops anterior?/posterior? and rightward?/leftward?

27. The heart tube loops anterior and leftward. This results in ventricular _____.

28. Septation of the heart is accomplished by three distinct mechanisms: 1.)_____, 2.)_____ and 3.)_____.

29. True or False: The atrioventricular valves are carved out of the internal layer of the ventricular muscular wall.

CHAPTER 2 (UNIT TWO) - BASIC EMBRYOLOGY

BOARD REVIEW QUESTIONS - Section 2A

1. The fetal heart tube appears by day:
   a. one
   b. seven
   c. fourteen
   d. twenty one

2. The heart is completely formed by week:
   a. one
   b. three
   c. five
   d. seven

3. The heart tube loops:
   a. anteriorly and leftward
   b. anteriorly and rightward
   c. posteriorly and leftward
   d. posteriorly and rightward

4. The looping of the heart tube creates the:
   a. bulbus cordis
   b. truncus arteriosus
   c. conus arteriosus
   d. bulboventricular loop

5. The junction between the primitive ventricle and the bulbus cordis is the:
   a. truncus arteriosus
   b. aortic sac
   c. bulboventricular foramen
   d. atrioventricular canal

6. Blood flow in the heart tube is directed:
   a. anteriorly
   b. posteriorly
   c. cephalad
   d. caudad

7. Which of the following contributes to the formation of the vena cava, coronary sinus and posterior walls of the right and left atrium?
   a. sinus venosus
   b. atrioventricular canal
   c. bulbus cordis
   d. truncus arteriosus

8. All of the following are associated with the development of the interatrial septum except:
    a. septum primum
    b. septum secundum
    c. foramen ovale
    d. trabecular septum

9. Which of the following divides the atrioventricular orifice in the fetal heart?
    a. muscular septum
    b. bulbus cordis
    c. septum primum
    d. endocardial cushions

10. The primitive ventricle is a usually a morphologic:
    a. right ventricle
    b. left ventricle
    c. anterior ventricle
    d. posterior ventricle

11. Which of the following contributes to the formation of the right ventricle, ventricular outflow tracts and truncus arteriosus?
    a. septum primum
    b. truncus arteriosus
    c. bulbus cordis
    d. atrioventricular canal

12. Which of the following contributes to the formation of the aortic and pulmonary trunks?
    a. bulbus cordis
    b. septum secundum
    c. truncus arteriosus
    d. endocardial cushions

13. The third aortic arch contributes to the formation of the:
    a. interatrial septum
    b. endocardial cushions
    c. ductus arteriosus
    d. internal carotid artery

14. The fourth aortic arch contributes to the formation of the:
    a. endocardial cushions
    b. bulbus cordis
    c. ductus arteriosus
    d. aortic arch

CHAPTER 2 (UNIT TWO) - BASIC EMBRYOLOGY

15. The sixth aortic arch contributes to the formation of all of the following except:
    a. internal carotid artery
    b. right pulmonary artery
    c. left pulmonary artery
    d. ductus arteriosus

16. The ascending aorta is derived from the:
    a. truncus arteriosus
    b. sinus venosus
    c. aortic sac
    d. fifth arch

17. Which of the following would be considered a cono-truncal abnormality?
    a. bicuspid aortic valve
    b. tetralogy of Fallot
    c. atrioventricular septal defect
    d. ventricular septal defect

18. The cardiac tube loops anterior and leftward. This results in:
    a. d-transposition of the great arteries
    b. l-transposition
    c. mitral atresia
    d. total anomalous pulmonary venous return

ANSWERS - Section 2A

Review practice answers

1. three
2. seven
3. anteriorly, right
4. bulboventricular
5. bulboventricular
6. sinus venosus, primitive atria, atrioventricular canal, primitive ventricle, bulbus cordis, truncus arteriosus, aortic sac, arches
7. sinus venosus
8. True
9. primitive atria
10. primum, secundum
11. foramen ovale
12. True
13. atrioventricular
14. endocardial
15. True
16. primitive ventricle
17. True
18. bulbus cordis
19. truncus arteriosus
20. True
21. 6
22. third
23. fourth
24. sixth
25. sac
26. anterior, rightward
27. inversion
28. passive, active, combination
29. True

Board review answers

1. d
2. d
3. b
4. d
5. c
6. c
7. a
8. d

9. d
10. b
11. c
12. c
13. d
14. d
15. a
16. c
17. b
18. b

CHAPTER 2 (UNIT TWO) - BASIC EMBRYOLOGY

FETAL CIRCULATION

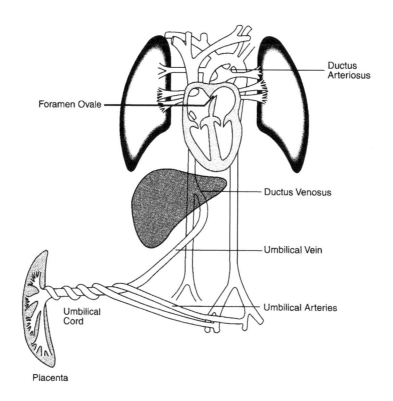

Ductus Arteriosus

Foramen Ovale

Ductus Venosus

Umbilical Vein

Umbilical Arteries

Umbilical Cord

Placenta

POSTNATAL CIRCULATION

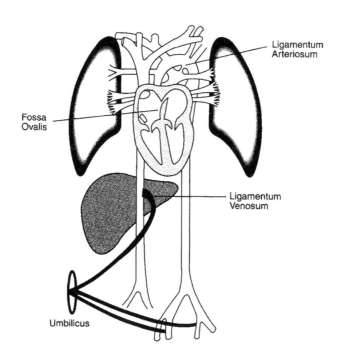

Ligamentum Arteriosum

Fossa Ovalis

Ligamentum Venosum

Umbilicus

CHAPTER 2 (UNIT TWO) - BASIC EMBRYOLOGY

Section 2B
Comparison of Fetal and Postnatal Circulation

1. FETAL CIRCULATION

Fetal circulation depends upon: the placental oxygenation of fetal blood, three intrafetal shunts, and the fetal heart to provide blood pressure.

Placental oxygenation

The fetal lungs are collapsed and possess high vascular resistance. Fetal blood is oxygenated in the placenta. Blood flow entering the placenta is poorly oxygenated, while blood flow leaving the placenta possesses the highest oxygen saturation in the fetal circulation.

Intrafetal circulatory shunts

Blood flow enters the fetus through the umbilical vein, passes through the ductus venosus (the first fetal shunt), largely avoiding flow through the liver, through the inferior vena cava (IVC) and into the right atrium. The blood flow entering the right atrium from the IVC is high in oxygen saturation. This IVC flow is preferentially directed by the eustachian valve through the foramen ovale (second fetal shunt). A portion of the blood flowing from the IVC is joined by blood flow from the superior vena cava (SVC) and the coronary sinus (CS). Both the blood from the SVC and CS are very desaturated.

These three streams jointly flow through the tricuspid valve, right ventricle, pulmonary valve and main pulmonary artery. The fetal lungs are collapsed and the pulmonary vasculature is highly resistant (high pulmonary vascular resistance) to flow. Only a small percentage of pulmonary blood flow enters the pulmonary vascular bed. Most pulmonary artery blood flow passes through the ductus arteriosus (third fetal shunt), and into the descending thoracic aorta.

The fetal heart

The blood flow from the IVC which passed through the foramen ovale into the left atrium is joined by desaturated blood returning from the lungs via the pulmonary veins. This blood passes through the mitral valve, left ventricle, aortic valve into the ascending aorta. It is the most highly oxygen saturated blood in the systemic arterial system. As this blood reaches the head, neck and arm vessels, the brain receives the most highly saturated blood available. The umbilical arteries carry the deoxygenated blood back to the maternal placenta.

2. POSTNATAL CIRCULATION

The three fetal circulatory shunts are: the foramen ovale, ductus arteriosus and the ductus venosus; all normally close after birth.

With birth, the lungs inflate, decreasing pulmonary vascular resistance and right heart pressures, while left heart pressures increase, resulting in closure of the foramen ovale which becomes the fossa ovalis in the adult.

The ductus arteriosus closes within 48 to 72 hours after birth due to the exposure of oxygenated blood coming from the now left to right shunt. The ductus arteriosus eventually becomes the ligamentum arteriosum. The ductus venosus closes due to a decrease in blood flow across the vessel and becomes the ligamentum venosum.

CHAPTER 2 (UNIT TWO) - BASIC EMBRYOLOGY

REVIEW PRACTICE - Section 2B

1. The oxygenation and exchange of carbon dioxide of fetal blood takes place in the maternal _____.

2. Oxygenated blood returns to the fetal heart via the umbilical _____.

3. The _____ _____ delivers blood from the umbilical vein to the inferior vena cava, thus bypassing the liver.

4. The _____ valve directs blood entering the right atrium to the foramen ovale.

5. True or False: In the fetal heart, the shunt between the atria is right to left.

6. The _____ _____ allows blood to be shunted from the pulmonary artery to the aorta in the fetal heart.

7. True or False: The shunt between the aorta and pulmonary artery in the fetus is right to left.

8. Deoxygenated blood returns to the placenta via the umbilical _____ in fetal circulation.

9. True or False: With birth, the lungs inflate, right atrial, right ventricular and pulmonary artery pressures decrease and left heart pressures increase.

10. The _____ _____ closes due to an increase in left atrial pressure.

11. True or False: The foramen ovale will become the fossa ovalis in the adult.

12. The _____ _____ closes upon birth due to an increase in oxygen content in the aorta.

13. The ductus arteriosus becomes the _____ _____ in the adult.

14. The _____ _____ closes due to a decrease in blood flow across the vessel, thus allowing blood flow to the liver.

15. The ductus venosus becomes the _____ _____ in the adult.

16. True or False: Blood enters the systemic arterial fetal system from two sources: the ductus arteriosus and the ascending aorta.

17. During fetal circulation the right ventricle pumps against a highly resistant pulmonary bed and arterial bed which means the fetal right ventricle will be thicker?/thinner? than the left ventricle.

18. True or False: During fetal circulation the right heart handles a larger volume of blood than the left heart.

19. True or False: During fetal circulation the left and right pulmonary arteries are relatively underdeveloped at birth due to the decrease in the flow volume of blood.

BOARD REVIEW QUESTIONS - Section 2B

1. Fetal blood oxygenation occurs in the maternal:
   a. heart
   b. lungs
   c. placenta
   d. aorta

2. Oxygenated blood returns to the fetal heart via the:
   a. umbilical artery
   b. umbilical vein
   c. maternal placenta
   d. fetal aorta

3. Which valve directs blood from the inferior vena cava to the foramen ovale in the fetal heart?
   a. tricuspid
   b. mitral
   c. thebesian
   d. eustachian

4. In the fetal heart, fetal blood at the atrial level is shunted right to left via the:
   a. foramen ovale
   b. ductus arteriosus
   c. ligamentum venosum
   d. ductus venosus

5. The vessel that shunts fetal blood right to left between the pulmonary artery and aorta is the:
   a. foramen ovale
   b. ductus arteriosus
   c. ligamentum arteriosum
   d. ductus venosus

6. Deoxygenated blood from the fetal heart returns to the maternal placenta via the:
   a. umbilical artery
   b. umbilical vein
   c. maternal placenta
   d. fetal aorta

7. All of the following are true statements concerning events that occur after birth except:
   a. systemic pressure increases
   b. pulmonary vascular resistance increases
   c. right heart pressures decrease
   d. foramen ovale closes

8. The foramen ovale closes after birth due to an increase in:
    a. right heart pressures
    b. left heart pressures
    c. pulmonary vascular resistance
    d. respirations

9. The ductus arteriosus closes due to increased:
    a. systemic pressure
    b. venous pressure
    c. respirations
    d. weight

10. The ductus venosus closes after birth and becomes the:
    a. ligamentum venosum
    b. ligamentum arteriosum
    c. umbilical ligament
    d. fossa ovalis

11. The umbilical artery after birth becomes the umbilical:
    a. artery
    b. vein
    c. ligament
    d. venosum

12. The umbilical vein after birth becomes the ligamentum:
    a. arteriosum
    b. venosum
    c. teres
    d. ovalis

13. The foramen ovale after birth becomes the:
    a. ligamentum arteriosum
    b. ligamentum venosum
    c. fossa ovalis
    d. ligamentum teres

14. The ductus arteriosus after birth becomes the:
    a. ligamentum arteriosum
    b. ligamentum venosum
    c. fossa ovalis
    d. ligamentum teres

15. All of the following are true statements concerning fetal circulation except:
    a. fetal right ventricle is thicker than the fetal left ventricle
    b. right heart handles a larger volume of blood than left heart
    c. pulmonary artery branches are underdeveloped at birth
    d. blood enters the systemic circulation only at the ductus arteriosus level

CHAPTER 2 (UNIT TWO) - BASIC EMBRYOLOGY

ANSWERS - Section 2B

Review practice answers

1. placenta
2. vein
3. ductus venosus
4. eustachian
5. True
6. ductus arteriosus
7. True
8. artery
9. True
10. foramen ovale
11. True
12. ductus arteriosus
13. ligamentum arteriosum
14. ductus venosus
15. ligamentum venosum
16. True
17. thicker
18. True
19. True

Board review answers

1. c
2. b
3. d
4. a
5. b
6. a
7. b
8. b
9. a
10. a
11. c
12. c
13. c
14. a
15. d

CHAPTER 2 (UNIT TWO) - BASIC EMBRYOLOGY

CHAPTER THREE
CONGENITAL DEFECTS

Section 3A
Abnormalities of Septation

Abnormalities of septation consist of atrial septal defects and ventricular septal defects.

Atrial Septal Defects

There are four types of atrial septal defects: ostium secundum, ostium primum, sinus venosus, and coronary sinus.

The ostium secundum is a defect involving the foramen ovale region of the interatrial septum. It is associated with mitral valve prolapse.

The ostium primum is a defect in the inferior area of the interatrial septum. It is associated with cleft atrioventricular valve.

The sinus venosus is a defect in the upper area of the interatrial septum, posterior to the fossa ovalis. It is associated with partial anomalous pulmonary venous return.

The coronary sinus is an uncommon atrial septal defect located inferior to the fossa ovalis where the coronary sinus enters the right atrium.

Ventricular Septal Defects

There are four ventricular septal defects: membraneous, trabecular, inlet, and outlet.

The membranous is a defect located below the aortic valve at the level of the left ventricular outflow tract.

The trabecular is a defect that may be located in different regions of the muscular ventricular septum. They can be multiple ("swiss-cheese"). May be referred to as muscular.

The inlet is a defect located posteriorly and inferiorly beneath the posterior tricuspid valve leaflet. It may also be referred to as posterior or AV canal type.

The outlet is a defect located in the right ventricular outflow tract inferior to the pulmonary valve. It may also be referred to as supulmonic or supracristal.

Section 3B
Abnormal Vasculature and Resulting Lesions

Coarctation is an abnormal narrowing of the descending thoracic aorta. Commonly associated with bicuspid aortic valve. (50%)

Tetralogy of Fallot is a lesion which consists of four components: aortic override, malalignment ventricular septal defect, subvalvular pulmonic stenosis and right ventricular hypertrophy.

Transposition of the great arteries is where the aorta originates from the right ventricle and the pulmonary artery originates from the left ventricle. Also called d-transposition.

Corrected transposition of the great arteries is a ventricular inversion with the aorta originating from the right ventricle and the pulmonary artery originating from the left ventricle. Also referred to as l-transposition.

Truncus arteriosus is a condition in which the coronary arteries, main pulmonary artery and aortic arch all arise from a common trunk (aorta).

Double outlet right ventricle is a condition in which the aorta and pulmonary artery both originate from the right ventricle. A malalignment ventricular septal defect is present.

Supravalvular aortic stenosis is an obstruction caused by narrowing of the aorta above the aortic valve.

Supravalvular pulmonic stenosis is an obstruction caused by narrowing of the pulmonary artery above the pulmonic valve.

Peripheral pulmonary stenosis is an obstruction due to abnormal narrowing of the distal pulmonary arteries.

Right aortic arch is a condition in which the aorta is located to the right of the trachea. Interrupted aortic arch is a lack of communication between the aortic arch and the descending thoracic aorta.

Vascular rings and double aortic arch is a ring formed around the trachea and esophagus due to the abnormal persistence of the aortic arches.

Total anomalous pulmonary venous return is a condition in which all four pulmonary veins connect to the right atrium via a common venous chamber or to a systemic vein.

Section 3C
Persistence of Normal Fetal Communication

Persistent fetal circulation is the failure of pulmonary vascular resistance to decrease after birth. This will cause the ductus arteriosus and patent foramen ovale to persist in shunting blood from right to left.

Patent foramen ovale is the failure of the foramen ovale to seal completely. This occurs in approximately 25% of adults. An increase in right heart pressures may result in paradoxical embolism through a patent foramen ovale.

Patent ductus arteriosus is the failure of the ductus arteriosus to close as it should shortly after birth, but may persist due to a variety of reasons including prematurity, maternal rubella and high altitude birth.

Section 3D
Valvular Anomalies

There are three types of atrioventricular septal defect: partial, complete and intermediate. Partial is an ostium primum atrial septal defect and cleft mitral valve. Complete is an ostium primum atrial septal defect, ventricular septal defect and common atrioventricular valve. Incomplete is two separate atrioventricular orifices, a left ventricular-right atrial shunt and three leaflets with a cleft of the left atrioventricular valve.

Valvular aortic stenosis is an abnormal narrowing due to fusion of the aortic valve cusps.

Bicuspid aortic valve is an aortic valve with two cusps and a raphe.

Valvular pulmonic stenosis is an abnormal narrowing of the pulmonic valve due to fusion of the pulmonic valve cusps.

Pulmonary atresia with an intact interventricular septum is the absence of the pulmonary valve with an underdeveloped right ventricle and intact interventricular septum.

Ebstein's anomaly is the abnormal displacement of the tricuspid valve towards the cardiac apex with atrialization of the right ventricle.

Uhl's anomaly is a right ventricular dilated cardiomyopathy due to fatty displacement of the right ventricular free wall.

Tricuspid atresia is a total absence of the tricuspid valve with hypoplasia of the right ventricle.

Mitral atresia is the total absence of the mitral valve, often associated with aortic valve atresia and hypoplasia of the the left ventricle. (hypoplastic left heart syndrome)

Cor triatriatum is a perforated membrane that partitions the left atrium. The insertion points of the membrane are located above the fossa ovalis.

Supravalvular mitral stenosis is an obstructive ridge or stenosing ring located just proximal to the mitral valve.

REVIEW PRACTICE - Sections 3A, 3B, 3C, 3D

1. The type of atrial septal defect that affects the central portion of the interatrial septum is called an _____ _____ atrial septal defect.

2. The atrial septal defect that affects the lower portion of the interatrial septum is:_____ _____.

3. The ostium primum atrial septal defect is associated with _____ mitral valve.

4. The atrial septal defect that affects the upper portion of the interatrial septum is called _____ _____.

5. The sinus venosus atrial septal defect is associated with _____ _____ pulmonary venous return.

6. True or False: The coronary sinus atrial septal defect is rare.

7. The ventricular septal defect that is located below the aortic valve is the _____ ventricular septal defect.

8. The _____ ventricular septal defect affects the muscular portion of the interventricular septum.

9. The _____ ventricular septal defect affects the posterior portion of the interventricular septum.

10. The _____ ventricular septal defect is located in the right ventricular outflow tract below the pulmonic valve.

11. _____ of the aorta is an abnormal narrowing of the descending thoracic aorta.

12. True or False: Bicuspid aortic valve is commonly associated with coarctation of the aorta.

13. The combination of aortic override, malalignment ventricular septal defect, subvalvular pulmonic stenosis and right ventricular hypertrophy is called _____ of _____.

14. _____ of the great arteries is present when the aorta originates from the right ventricle and the pulmonary artery originates from the left ventricle.

15. _____ transposition of the great arteries is ventricular inversion with the aorta originating from the right ventricle and the pulmonary artery from the left ventricle.

16. _____ _____ is a single artery overriding a malalignment ventricular septal defect with the pulmonary artery, coronary arteries and arch vessels originating from the single great vessel.

17. In _____ _____ right ventricle, the aorta and pulmonary both originate from the right ventricle.

18. _____ aortic stenosis is an abnormal narrowing of the aorta above the aortic valve.

19. _____ pulmonic stenosis is the abnormal narrowing of the pulmonary artery above the pulmonic valve.

20. _____ pulmonary stenosis is the abnormal narrowing of the pulmonary artery branches.

21. Pulmonary _____ is the absence of the pulmonary valve with hypolasia of the right ventricle.

22. In a _____ aortic arch, the aorta is to the right of the trachea.

23. In _____ aortic arch, there is a lack of communication between the aortic arch and the descending thoracic aorta.

24. In _____ ring and _____ aortic arch, a ring is formed around the trachea and esophagus due to the abnormal persistence of the aortic arches.

25. In _____ anomalous pulmonary venous return all four pulmonary veins connect to the right atrium.

26. Persistent _____ _____ is a right to left shunt of the foramen ovale and ductus arteriosus due to pulmonary hypertension.

27. Patent _____ _____ is the failure of the foramen ovale to seal completely.

28. Patent _____ _____ is present when the vessel between the aorta and pulmonary artery remains open after birth.

29. An ostium primum atrial septal defect combined with cleft mitral valve is a _____ atrioventricular septal defect.

30. An ostium primum atrial septal defect, ventricular septal defect and a common atrioventricular valve is a _____ atrioventricular septal defect.

31. Valvular _____ stenosis is an abnormal narrowing of the aortic valve due to fusion of the aortic valve cusps.

32. An aortic valve with two cusps and a raphe is called a _____ aortic valve.

33. Valvular _____ stenosis is the abnormal narrowing of the pulmonic valve due to fusion of the pulmonic valve.

34. The displacement of the tricuspid valve abnormally downwards with atrialization of the right ventricle is _____ anomaly.

35. A type of right ventricular dilated cardiomyopathy where there is fatty displacement of the right ventricular free wall is called _____ anomaly.

36. _____ atresia is total absence of the tricuspid valve with right ventricular hypoplasia.

37. _____ atresia is total absence of the mitral valve with left ventricular hypoplasia.

38. The combination of mitral valve atresia, aortic valve atresia, and hypoplasia of the left ventricle is called _____ left heart syndrome.

39. In _____ _____ an obstructing membrane partitions the left atrium.

40. An obstructive ridge or stenosing ring located just proximal to the mitral valve is called _____ mitral stenosis.

BOARD REVIEW QUESTIONS - Sections 3A, 3B, 3C, 3D

1. The atrial septal defect that involves the central region of the interatrial septum is called the:
    a. ostium primum
    b. ostium secundum
    c. sinus venosus
    d. coronary sinus

2. The atrial septal defect that affects the lower portion of the interatrial septum is called the:
    a. ostium primum
    b. ostium secundum
    c. sinus venosus
    d. coronary sinus

3. Which of the following is most often associated with ostium primum atrial septal defect?
    a. bicuspid aortic valve
    b. trabecular ventricular septal defect
    c. cleft atrioventricular valve
    d. coarctation of the aorta

4. The atrial septal defect that affects the posterior region of the interatrial septum is called the:
    a. ostium secundum
    b. ostium primum
    c. sinus venosus
    d. coronary sinus

5. Which of the following findings is commonly associated with sinus venosus atrial septal defect?
    a. coarctation of the aorta
    b. bicuspid aortic valve
    c. malalignment ventricular septal defect
    d. anomalous pulmonary venous return

6. The ventricular septal defect that is located below the aortic valve is the:
    a. perimembranous
    b. trabecular
    c. outlet
    d. inlet

7. The ventricular septal defect that affects the trabecular interventricular septum is the:
    a. perimembranous
    b. muscular
    c. outlet
    d. inlet

8. The ventricular septal defect that affects the posterior portion of the interventricular septum is the:
    a. perimembranous
    b. trabecular
    c. outlet
    d. inlet

9. The ventricular septal defect that is located below the pulmonic valve is the:
    a. perimembranous
    b. trabecular
    c. inlet
    d. outlet

10. The abnormal narrowing of the descending thoracic aorta is called:
    a. coarctation
    b. transposition
    c. tetralogy
    d. malalignment

11. Which of the following is most commonly associated with coarctation of the aorta?
    a. ostium primum atrial septal defect
    b. bicuspid aortic valve
    c. mitral valve prolapse
    d. outlet ventricular septal defect

12. All of the following are considered a primary component of tetralogy of Fallot except:
    a. pulmonic stenosis
    b. malalignment ventricular septal defect
    c. left ventricular hypertrophy
    d. aortic override

13. The aorta originates from the right ventricle and the pulmonary artery originates from the left ventricle. This is called:
    a. tetralogy of Fallot
    b. simple transposition of the great arteries
    c. corrected transposition of the great arteries
    d. double outlet right ventricle

14. Which of the following is associated with ventricular inversion?
    a. simple transposition of the great arteries
    b. corrected transposition of the great arteries
    c. double outlet right ventricle
    d. tricuspid atresia

15. Which of the following is defined as a single artery with a malalignment ventricular septal defect?
    a. truncus arteriosus
    b. tetralogy of Fallot
    c. simple transposition of the great arteries
    d. coarctation

16. The aorta and pulmonary both originate from the right ventricle. This is called:
    a. tetralogy of Fallot
    b. truncus arteriosus
    c. double outlet right ventricle
    d. d-transposition

17. All of the following may be considered right heart outflow tract obstructions except:
    a. supravalvular pulmonic stenosis
    b. peripheral pulmonary stenosis
    c. infundibular pulmonic stenosis
    d. tricuspid valve atresia

18. Which of the following is associated with a right to left shunt at the level of the foramen ovale and patent ductus arteriosus due to elevated pulmonary artery pressures?
    a. coarctation
    b. tetralogy of Fallot
    c. persistent fetal circulation
    d. truncus arteriosus

19. Failure of the flap to seal completely between the two atria is called:
    a. persistent ductus arteriosus
    b. patent foramen ovale
    c. ligamentum arteriosum
    d. peristent fetal circulation

20. The communication between the aorta and pulmonary artery that may persist after birth is called:
    a. patent foramen ovale
    b. patent ductus arteriosus
    c. ligamentum arteriosum
    d. persistent fetal circulation

21. A partial atrioventricular septal defect is the combination of which pathologies?
    a. mitral valve prolapse, secundum atrial septal defect
    b. sinus venosus atrial septal defect, partial anomalous pulmonary venous return
    c. ostium primum atrial septal defect, cleft mitral valve
    d. coronary sinus atrial septal defect, persistent left superior vena cava

22. The combination of ostium primum atrial septal defect, ventricular septal defect and common atrioventricular valve is called:
    a. truncus arteriosus
    b. complete atrioventricular septal defect
    c. tetralogy of Fallot
    d. double outlet right ventricle

23. The abnormal insertion of the tricuspid valve downward with atrialization of the right ventricle is known as:
    a. cleft tricuspid valve
    b. tricuspid atresia
    c. Ebstein's anomaly
    d. tricuspid valve prolapse

24. A right ventricular dilated cardiomyopathy where there is displacement of the right ventricular free wall with fatty tissue is called:
    a. Ebstein's anomaly
    b. Uhl's anomaly
    c. d-transposition
    d. l-transposition

25. Total absence of the pulmonary valve is referred to as:
    a. atresia
    b. hypoplasia
    c. stenotic
    d. regurgitant

26. Total absence of the mitral valve or tricuspid valve is referred to as:
    a. regurgitant
    b. stenotic
    c. hypoplastic
    d. atresia

27. An obstructing membrane which partitions the left atrium is called:
    a. cor triatriatum
    b. discrete subaortic stenosis
    c. partial anomalous pulmonary venous return
    d. mitral valve atresia

ANSWERS - Sections 3A, 3B, 3C, 3D

Review practice answers

1. ostium secundum
2. ostium primum
3. cleft
4. sinus venosus
5. partial anomalous
6. True
7. membranous
8. trabecular
9. inlet
10. outlet
11. coarctation
12. True
13. tetralogy of Fallot
14. d-transposition
15. (l) corrected
16. truncus arteriosus
17. double outlet
18. supravalvular
19. supravalvular
20. peripheral
21. atresia
22. right
23. interrupted
24. vascular, double
25. total
26. fetal circulation
27. foramen ovale
28. ductus arteriosus
29. partial
30. complete
31. aortic
32. bicuspid
33. pulmonic
34. Ebstein's
35. Uhl's
36. tricuspid
37. mitral
38. hypoplastic
39. cor triatriatum
40. supravalvular

CHAPTER 3 (UNIT THREE) - CONGENITAL DEFECTS

Board review answers

1. b
2. a
3. c
4. c
5. d
6. a
7. b
8. d
9. d
10. a
11. b
12. c
13. b
14. b
15. a
16. c
17. d
18. c
19. b
20. b
21. c
22. b
23. c
24. b
25. a
26. d
27. a

CHAPTER 3 (UNIT THREE) - CONGENITAL DEFECTS

CHAPTER FOUR
CARDIAC PHYSIOLOGY

SECTION 4A
Electrophysiology and the Conduction System

1. PROPAGATION OF ELECTRICAL ACTIVITY

The electrical conduction system initiates and maintains rhythmic contraction of the heart. The cardiac conduction system is composed of the following: sinoatrial (SA) node, internodal pathways, atrioventricular (AV) node, bundle of His, bundle branches, and Purkinje fibers.

Sinoatrial (SA) node: The SA node is considered the pacemaker of the heart because its intrinsic firing rate (rate of depolarization) is the fastest (most automatic) of the heart.

The SA node is located in the upper wall of the right atrium near the entrance of the superior vena cava. The SA node fires electrical impulses 60 to 100 times per minute.

Internodal tracts: The cardiac impulse is carried to both atria by way of the internodal tracts which causes the atria to depolarize and then contract. The tract that delivers the impulse to the left atrium is called Bachmann's bundle.

Atrioventricular (AV) node: The AV node delays the electrical impulse 0.10 second before delivering the impulse to the bundle of His. The AV node is located at the floor of the right atrium near the interatrial septum.

Bundle of His: The bundle of His is a thin bundle which connects the AV node to the bundle branches. The bundle of His is a potential pacemaker site with an automatic firing rate of between 40 and 60 beats per minute.

Right and left bundle branches: The right bundle branch runs along the right side of the interventricular septum and delivers the electrical impulse to the right ventricle. The left bundle branch runs along the left side of the interventricular septum and delivers the electrical impulse to the left ventricle. Normally the left ventricle depolarizes slightly before the right ventricle.

Purkinje fibers: The bundle branches terminate in a network of fibers called the Purkinje fibers which are located in both the right and left ventricles. The cardiac impulse travels to the Purkinje fibers which causes ventricular depolarization and then ventricular contraction. The Purkinje fibers have an automatic firing rate of between 20 and 40 beats per minute.

The electrical activity that is generated and spread throughout the heart creates an electrical change in each cardiac cell. This electrical activity of the heart can be monitored and measured on an electrocardiogram.

Associated terms

Automaticity:	The heart can begin and maintain rhythmic activity without the aid of the nervous system.
Excitability:	Cardiac muscle can accept and respond to electrical impulses.
Conductivity:	A cardiac cell can transfer an electrical impulse to a neighboring cardiac cell.
Contractility:	The heart responds to an electrical impulse by contracting.

CHAPTER 4 (UNIT FOUR) - CARDIAC PHYSIOLOGY

REVIEW PRACTICE - Section 4A

1. The seven components of the cardiac conduction system are: 1. _____node, 2. _____ pathways, 3. _____ node, 4. _____ of _____, 5. _____ bundle branch, 6._____ bundle branch, and the 7. _____

2. True or False: The right coronary artery supplies oxygenated blood to the sinoatrial (SA) and atrioventricular (AV) nodes.

3. The _____ node is considered the pacemaker of the heart.

4. True or False: The sinoatrial node is commonly referred to as the SA node.

5. True or False: The sinoatrial node is located in the upper wall of the right atrium near the entrance of the superior vena cava.

6. The sinoatrial (SA) node fires electrical impulses normally at a rate of between _____ to _____ times per minute.

7. The _____ tracts deliver the electrical impulse from the sinoatrial node to the atria.

8. The _____ bundle is a well formed internodal tract that delivers the electrical impulse from the sinoatrial node to the left atrium.

9. The _____ node delays the electrical impulse 0.10 second before delivering the impulse to the bundle of His.

10. True or False: The atrioventricular node is commonly referred to as the AV node.

11. True or False: The atrioventricular node is located at the floor of the right atrium near the interatrial septum.

12. The bundle of _____ is a thin bundle which connects the atrioventricular node to the bundle branches.

13. The right and _____ bundle branches deliver the electrical impulse to the ventricles.

14. The _____ fibers deliver the electrical impulse from the bundle branches to the ventricular walls causing ventricular depolarization and ventricular contraction.

15. The automatic firing rate for the SA node is between _____ to _____ beats per minute.

16. The automatic firing rate for the His bundle is between _____ and _____ beats per minute.

17. The automatic firing rate for the Purkinje fibers is between _____ and _____beats per minute.

18. The _____ records the electrical activity of the heart.

19. _____ infers that the heart can begin and maintain rhythmic activity without the aid of the nervous system.

20. _____ means that cardiac muscle cells can accept and respond to electrical impulses.

21. _____ means that a cardiac cell is able to transfer an electrical impulse to a neighboring cardiac cell.

22. _____ means that the heart responds to an electrical impulse by contracting.

CHAPTER 4 (UNIT FOUR) - CARDIAC PHYSIOLOGY

BOARD REVIEW QUESTIONS - Section 4A

1. All of the following are components of the cardiac conduction system except:
   a. sinoatrial node
   b. internodal tracts
   c. interatrial septum
   d. atrioventricular node

2. Which coronary artery supplies oxygenated blood to the sinoatrial node and the atrioventricular node?
   a. left main
   b. left anterior descending
   c. circumflex
   d. right coronary artery

3. Which of the following components of the cardiac conduction system is considered the pacemaker of the heart?
   a. sinoatrial node
   b. internodal tracts
   c. atrioventricular node
   d. bundle of His

4. The sinoatrial node is located closest to the:
   a. superior vena cava
   b. inferior vena cava
   c. coronary sinus
   d. right coronary artery

5. The sinoatrial node normally fires electrical impulses at a rate of:
   a. 60 to 100 per minute
   b. 40 to 60 per minute
   c. 20 to 40 per minute
   d. 10 to 20 per minute

6. The His bundle has an automatic firing rate of between:
   a. 60 to 100 per minute
   b. 40 to 60 per minute
   c. 20 to 40 per minute
   d. 0 to 10 per minute

7. The Purkinje fibers have an automatic firing rate of between:
   a. 0 to 10 per minute
   b. 20 to 40 per minute
   c. 40 to 60 per minute
   d. 60 to 100 per minute

8. Which of the following components of the cardiac conduction system delivers the electrical impulse from the sinoatrial node to the atria?
    a. internodal tracts
    b. atrioventricular node
    c. bundle of His
    d. bundle branches

9. Which of the following deliver the electrical impulse from the sinoatrial node to the left atrium?
    a. Bachmann's
    b. Bernoulli's
    c. Wenkebach
    d. His

10. Which of the following components of the cardiac conduction system deliver the electrical impulse to the bundle of His after a 0.10 second delay?
    a. sinoatrial node
    b. internodal tracts
    c. atrioventricular node
    d. bundle of His

11. The atrioventricular node is located at the floor of the:
    a. left atrium
    b. right atrium
    c. right ventricle
    d. left ventricle

12. Which of the following components of the cardiac conduction system deliver the electrical impulse from the atrioventricular node to the bundle branches?
    a. internodal tracts
    b. atrioventricular node
    c. bundle of His
    d. Purkinje fibers

13. Which of the following components of the cardiac conduction system delivers the electrical impulse from the bundle of His to the ventricles?
    a. sinoatrial node
    b. internodal tracts
    c. His bundle
    d. right/left bundle branches

14. Which of the following components of the cardiac conduction system delivers the electrical impulse from the bundle branches to the ventricular walls?
    a. sinoatrial node
    b. atrioventricular node
    c. bundle of His
    d. Purkinje fibers

15. Which of the following terms means the heart can begin and maintain rhythmic activity without the aid of the nervous system?
    a. automaticity
    b. excitabilty
    c. conductivity
    d. contractility

16. Which of the following terms means that cardiac muscle can accept and respond to electrical impulses?
    a. automaticity
    b. excitability
    c. conductivity
    d. contractility

17. Which of the following terms means that a cardiac cell is able to transfer an electrical impulse to a neighboring cardiac cell?
    a. automaticity
    b. excitability
    c. conductivity
    d. contractility

18. Which of the following terms means that the heart responds to an electrical impulse by contracting?
    a. automaticity
    b. excitability
    c. conductivity
    d. contractility

ANSWERS - Section 4A

Review practice answers

1. sinoatrial (SA), internodal, atrioventricular (AV), bundle His, right, left, Purkinje fibers
2. True
3. sinoatrial (SA)
4. True
5. True
6. 60, 100
7. internodal
8. Bachmann's
9. atrioventricular (AV)
10. True
11. True
12. His
13. left
14. Purkinje
15. 60, 100
16. 40, 60
17. 20, 40
18. electrocardiogram
19. automaticity
20. excitability
21. conductivity
22. contractility

Board review answers

1. c
2. d
3. a
4. a
5. a
6. b
7. b
8. a
9. a
10. c
11. b
12. c
13. d
14. d
15. a
16. b
17. c
18. d

2. EXCITATION CONTRACTION COUPLING

Each cardiac cell is bathed by positively and negatively charged electrolytes. These electrolytes cause the resting cardiac cell to have a net negative charge of -90 millivolts. This causes the cardiac cell to be in a polarized state and is called the resting membrane potential. When an electrical impulse is applied to the cardiac cell a threshold potential has been achieved and an action potential has been created. This action potential allows cardiac cell channels or gates to open and allow intracellular and extracellular electrolytes to be exchanged. This exchange of electrolytes is referred to as depolarization. Recovery from the depolarized state is called repolarization.

The action potential curve depicts the electrical activity of the cardiac cell over time. The curve demonstrates the action potential for the fast response cardiac cells such as the atrial and myocardial cells and the Purkinje fibers. The action potential curve has phases 0 through 4.

Phase 0 to 1: Cardiac cell rapid depolarization. Sodium rapidly enters the cell and potassium leaves the cell.

Phase 1: Early rapid repolarization. Potassium begins to reenter the cell as sodium leaves the cell.

Phase 2: Known as the plateau phase, it marks the point at which calcium enters the cardiac cell, causing cardiac cell contraction. This is the central component of the excitation-contraction coupling mechanism. Phase 2 coincides with the ST segment of the electrocardiogram.

Phase 3: Final rapid repolarization. The cell repolarizes by pumping sodium and calcium out while potassium is returning to the cell.

Phase 4: Resting phase. Sodium and calcium remain outside the cell while potassium remains inside the cell.

Important Facts:

Absolute refractory period: During phase 1 and 2, the cardiac cell will not respond to another stimulus, no matter how strong.

Relative refractory period: During phase 2 and 3, the cardiac cell can be stimulated again but the stimulus must be stronger than usual.

It is important to note that normally electrical events briefly precede mechanical events.

ACTION POTENTIAL CURVE

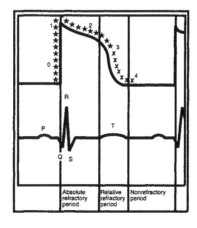

CHAPTER 4 (UNIT FOUR) - CARDIAC PHYSIOLOGY

REVIEW PRACTICE - Section 4A

1. The _____ potential curve depicts the electrical activity of the cardiac cell over time.

2. For the action potential curve, phase _____ to _____ marks cardiac cell rapid depolarization.

3. During rapid repolarization _____ rapidly enters the cardiac cell and _____ leaves the cell.

4. For the action potential curve, phase _____ marks early rapid repolarization.

5. True or False: During early rapid repolarization potassium reenters the cardiac cell while sodium leaves the cell.

6. For the action potential curve, phase _____ marks actual cardiac contraction.

7. True or False: The central component of the excitation-contraction coupling mechanism is the influx of calcium into the cardiac cell.

8. True or False: Calcium is important in causing cardiac cell contraction.

9. Phase two of the action potential curve closely coincides with the _____ segment of the electrocardiogram.

10. For the action potential curve, phase _____ represents final rapid repolarization.

11. True or False: During final rapid repolarization the cardiac cell repolarizes by pumping sodium and calcium out while potassium returns.

12. For the action potential curve, phase _____ represents the resting phase.

13. True or False: During the resting phase sodium and calcium remain outside the cell while potassium remains inside.

14. The _____ refractory period refers to the period where the cardiac cell will not respond to any stimulus no matter how strong.

15. The _____ refractory period refers to the point in the action potential curve where the cardiac cell will only respond to a very strong stimulus.

16. True or False: In the heart, electrical events precede mechanical events.

BOARD REVIEW QUESTIONS - Section 4A

1. Which of the following depicts the electrical activity of the cardiac cell over time?
   a. Wiggers diagram
   b. action potential curve
   c. pressure waveforms
   d. electrocardiogram

2. For the action potential curve, which of the following phases represent initial cardiac cell depolarization?
   a. 0 to 1
   b. 2
   c. 3
   d. 4

3. For the action potential curve, which phase represents a brief period of repolarization?
   a. 0 to 1
   b. 1
   c. 2
   d. 3

4. For the action potential curve, which phase represents actual cardiac contraction?
   a. 0 to 1
   b. 2
   c. 3
   d. 4

5. Which ion is important in causing actual cardiac contraction?
   a. calcium
   b. potassium
   c. sodium
   d. nitrogen

6. For the action potential curve, which phase represents repolarization?
   a. 0 to 1
   b. 2
   c. 3
   d. 4

7. For the action potential curve, which phase represents the resting state of the heart?
   a. 1
   b. 2
   c. 3
   d. 4

8. For the action potential curve, the period of titme where a cardiac cell will not accept a stimulus, no matter how strong the stimulus, is called:
    a. absolute refractory
    b. relative refractory
    c. pulse repetition
    d. isovolumic

9. For the action potential curve, the period of time where the cardiac cell can be stimulated but only by a very strong stimulus, is called:
    a. absolute refractory
    b. relative refractory
    c. pulse repetition
    d. isovolumic

10. Which of the following statements concerning the relationship between mechanical and electrical cardiac events is true?
    a. electrical follows mechanical
    b. mechanical precedes electrical
    c. electrical precedes mechanical
    d. electrical and mechanical occur simultaneously

11. According to the electrocardiogram, actual ventricular contraction coincides with the:
    a. P wave
    b. QRS complex
    c. ST segment
    d. T wave

CHAPTER 4 (UNIT FOUR) - CARDIAC PHYSIOLOGY

ANSWERS - Section 4A

Review practice answers

1. action
2. 0, 1
3. sodium, potassium
4. 1
5. True
6. 2
7. True
8. True
9. ST
10. 3
11. True
12. 4
13. True
14. absolute
15. relative
16. True

Board review answers

1. b
2. a
3. b
4. b
5. a
6. c
7. d
8. a
9. b
10. c
11. c

SECTION 4B
Mechanical Considerations and Events

1. FRANK - STARLING LAW

The Frank-Starling law of the heart states that the greater the stretch of the cardiac muscle cell (length or preload), the greater the force of contraction (tension) .

Preload is the length to which a cardiac myofibril is stretched prior to the next contraction. Since it is impossible to measure the length of a ventricular myocardial fibril clinically, preload is defined hemodynamically as the volume or pressure that exists in the ventricles at end-diastole. For the left heart, this is often described as left ventricular filling pressure and is measured hemodynamically as pulmonary artery wedge pressure. The pulmonary wedge pressure also reflects the pressure in the left atrium. For the right heart, right ventricular filling pressure is reflected by right atrial pressure or central venous pressure.

According to the Frank-Starling law, an increase in preload will lead to an increase in cardiac contraction and therefore an increase in cardiac performance (e.g. increased stroke volume, cardiac output). There is a limit to the law, with excessive myocardial fiber stretching leading to an actual reduction in the force of contraction and resultant ventricular failure.

The Frank-Starling law assures that the output of both ventricles will be equal. For example, an increase in venous return will result in an increase in right ventricular end-diastolic volume, force of contraction and stroke volume. This will lead to a balancing of output because there will be an increase in left ventricular end-diastolic volume, force of left ventricular contraction and stroke volume.

Conditions that increase ventricular preload include atrioventricular valve regurgitation, semilunar valve regurgitation, and congenital heart defect shunts.

STARLINGS CURVE

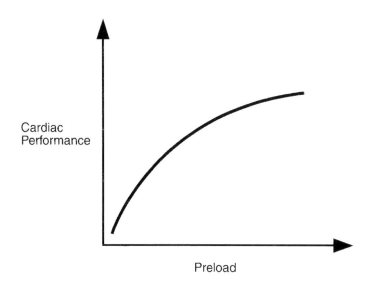

REVIEW PRACTICE - Section 4B

1. The _____ - _____ law of the heart states that the greater the stretch of the cardiac muscle cell (preload), the greater the force of contraction.

2. True or False: The Frank-Starling law may also be referred to as the length-tension relationship.

3. True or False: For the term length-tension relationship, length refers to the length the cardiac muscle cell is stretched.

4. True or False: For the term length-tension relationship, tension refers to cardiac contraction.

5. True or False: Preload is the length the cardiac cell is stretched prior to the next cardiac contraction.

6. True or False: It is difficult to directly measure the actual length of the cardiac cell clinically.

7. The pulmonary artery wedge pressure is an indirect measurement of _____ atrial and left ventricular diastolic pressure.

8. The central venous pressure is a measure of right heart?/left heart? filling pressures.

9. True or False: According to the Frank-Starling law of the heart, an increase in preload will lead to an increase in the strength of ventricular contraction.

10. True or False: There is a limit to Starling's law, with excessive myocardial fiber stretching leading to an actual reduction in the strength of cardiac contraction.

11. Mitral regurgitation will increase?/decrease? left heart preload.

12. Tricuspid regurgitation will increase?/decrease? right heart preload.

13. Aortic regurgitation will increase?/decrease? left heart preload.

14. Pulmonic valve regurgitation will increase?/decrease? right heart preload.

15. Atrial septal defect will increase?/decrease? right heart preload.

16. Ventricular septal defect will increase?/decrease? left heart preload.

17. Patent ductus arteriosus will increase?/decrease? left heart preload.

18. True or False: The vena cava and pulmonary veins would be considered preload vessels.

BOARD REVIEW QUESTIONS - Section 4B

1. Which of the following states that the greater the stretch of the cardiac muscle cell, the greater the force of contraction.
    a. Bernoulli
    b. Doppler
    c. Frank-Starling
    d. Bernheim

2. The Frank-Starling law may also be referred to as the:
    a. length-tension relationship
    b. force-velocity relationship
    c. interval-strength relationship
    d. isovolumic contraction relationship

3. The word length in length-tension relationship refers to cardiac:
    a. diastole
    b. diastasis
    c. cell stretch
    d. systole

4. The word tension in length-tension relationship refers to cardiac:
    a. diastole
    b. diastasis
    c. contraction
    d. cell stretch

5. Which of the following terms is defined as the length the cardiac cell is stretched prior to the next cardiac contraction?
    a. afterload
    b. preload
    c. noload
    d. sumload

6. The pulmonary artery wedge pressure reflects:
    a. left atrial pressure
    b. right atrial pressure
    c. pulmonary artery pressure
    d. right ventricular pressure

7. The central venous pressure reflects the pressure in the:
    a. right atrium
    b. left atrium
    c. left ventricle
    d. pulmonary artery

8. What effect will an increase in preload have on the force of ventricular contraction?
    a. decrease
    b. increase
    c. no change
    d. cannot be predicted

9. All of the following will increase preload of the left heart except:
    a. aortic regurgitation
    b. mitral regurgitation
    c. patent ductus arteriosus
    d. aortic stenosis

10. All of the following conditions will increase right heart preload except:
    a. tricuspid regurgitation
    b. pulmonary regurgitation
    c. ventricular septal defect
    d. atrial septal defect

11. According to Starling's law of the heart, significant mitral regurgitation initially will have which effect on left ventricular performance?
    a. enhance
    b. decrease
    c. varies
    d. cannot be predicted

ANSWERS - Section 4B

Review practice answers

1. Frank-Starling
2. True
3. True
4. True
5. True
6. True
7. left
8. right heart
9. True
10. True
11. increase
12. increase
13. increase
14. increase
15. increase
16. increase
17. increase
18. True

Board review answers

1. c
2. a
3. c
4. c
5. b
6. a
7. a
8. b
9. d
10. c
11. a

2. FORCE - VELOCITY RELATIONSHIP

Force refers to the load production that the myocardial fiber must produce. Velocity relates to the rate of myocardial fiber shortening during ventricular systole.

The greater the force the myocardial fiber must produce, the slower the rate of fiber shortening. Greater force is needed when the ventricle pumps against a higher resistance such as in valvular aortic stenosis. The term used to describe the resistance a ventricle faces during ejection is afterload. An increase in afterload means that the ventricle must produce a greater force which leads to a decrease in the rate of fiber shortening and cardiac performance. A reduction in afterload means a reduction in force and an increase in the rate of fiber shortening and an improvement in cardiac performance. Afterload is determined by arterial blood pressure, semilunar valve characteristics and blood viscosity.

Pathologies that increase afterload:

    Valvular aortic/pulmonic stenosis
    Subvalvular aortic/pulmonic stenosis
    Supravalvular aortic/pulmonic stenosis
    Systemic/pulmonary hypertension
    Coarctation of the aorta
    Renal artery stenosis

AFTERLOAD

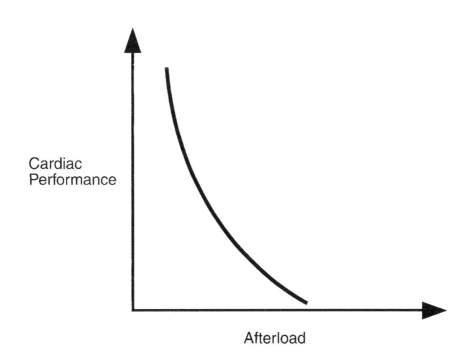

CHAPTER 4 (UNIT FOUR) - CARDIAC PHYSIOLOGY

REVIEW PRACTICE - Section 4B

1. _____ refers to the load production that the myocardial fibers must produce during ventricular systole.

2. _____ refers to the rate of myocardial fiber shortening during ventricular systole.

3. True or False: The force the myocardial fibers must produce is inversely related to the rate of fiber shortening.

4. True or False: The greater the force the myocardial fiber must produce, the slower the rate of fiber shortening.

5. _____ means the resistance or impedance the ventricle faces as it contracts.

6. True or False: An increase in afterload will mean an increase in myocardial load production and a decrease in the rate of fiber shortening and cardiac performance.

7. True or False: A reduction in afterload means a reduction in force and an increase in the rate of fiber shortening and cardiac performance.

8. True or False: An increase in afterload is associated with a decrease in cardiac performance.

9. True or False: A reduction in afterload generally will improve cardiac performance.

10. Afterload is dependent upon arterial _____ pressure, semilunar _____ characteristics and blood _____.

Tell if the following pathologies increase or decrease afterload:

11. _____Valvular aortic/pulmonic stenosis

12. _____Subvalvular aortic/pulmonic stenosis

13. _____Supravalvular aortic/pulmonic stenosis

14. _____Coarctation of the aorta

15. _____Systemic/pulmonary hypertension

16. True or False: The pulmonary artery and aorta would be considered afterload vessels.

BOARD REVIEW QUESTIONS - Section 4B

1. Which of the following refers to the load production that the myocardium must produce during ventricular systole?
   a. force
   b. velocity
   c. preload
   d. systole

2. Which of the following terms refers to the rate of myocardial fiber shortening?
   a. force
   b. velocity
   c. preload
   d. systole

3. Force and velocity are
   a. porportional
   b. directly related
   c. inversely related
   d. unrelated

4. With an increase in force, the velocity of fiber shortening will:
   a. increase
   b. decrease
   c. varies
   d. cannot be predicted

5. With a decrease in force, the velocity of fiber shortening will:
   a. increase
   b. decrease
   c. remain unchanged
   d. cannot be determined

6. Which of the following terms refers to the resistance a ventricle faces during ejection?
   a. afterload
   b. velocity
   c. diastole
   d. systole

7. What effect will an increase in afterload have on myocardial force?
   a. increase
   b. decrease
   c. no change
   d. cannot be predicted

8. What effect will an increase in afterload have on myocardial fiber shortening velocity?
    a. increase
    b. decrease
    c. no change
    d. cannot be predicted

9. What effect will an increase of afterload have on cardiac performance?
    a. increase
    b. decrease
    c. no change
    d. undetermined

10. Which of the following statements is true concerning valvular aortic stenosis?
    a. increase in ventricular force, velocity and afterload
    b. decrease in ventricular force, velocity and afterload
    c. increase in ventricular force, decrease in velocity and an increase in afterload
    d. decrease in ventricular force, increase in velocity and an increase in afterload

ANSWERS - Section 4B

Review practice answers

1. force
2. velocity
3. True
4. True
5. afterload
6. True
7. True
8. True
9. True
10. blood, valve, viscosity
11. increase
12. increase
13. increase
14. increase
15. increase
16. True

Board review answers

1. a
2. b
3. c
4. b
5. a
6. a
7. a
8. b
9. b
10. c

3. INTERVAL-STRENGTH RELATIONSHIP

The time interval between each heart beat and the strength of each ventricular contraction are directly related. As the interval between each heart beat increases, the strength of ventricular contraction will also increase. The primary example of this relationship is post-premature ventricular contraction. Immediately following the premature ventricular beat there is a compensatory pause, the interval between heart beats is increased, and the strength of the next ventricular contraction is increased. This phenomenon may also be referred to as post extra-systolic potentiation.

The sonographer may observe the interval-strength relationship graphically when examining a patient with valvular aortic stenosis or hypertrophic obstructive cardiomyopathy. Following a premature ventricular contraction and a compensatory pause, the peak velocity and peak pressure gradient will be increased in these patients.

REVIEW PRACTICE - Section 4B

1. The term _____ in interval-strength relationship refers to the time between each heart beat.

2. The term _____ in interval-strength refers to the ventricular systolic contraction strength.

3. True or False: In general, as the interval between each heart beat increases, the strength of ventricular contraction increases.

4. A _____ pause may immediately follow a premature ventricular contraction (PVC).

5. True or False: According to the interval-strength relationship, the heart beat that immediately follows a compensatory pause will be increased in strength.

6. The phenomenon where there is an increase in the strength of ventricular contraction following a premature ventricular contraction is called post extra-systolic _____.

7. True or False: According to the interval-strength relationship, the peak velocity across a stenotic aortic valve will be increased post premature ventricular contraction.

8. True or False: According to the interval-strength relationship, the peak velocity in a patient with hypertrophic obstructive cardiomyopathy will be increased post premature ventricular contraction.

9. True or False: According to the interval-strength relationship, the peak systolic velocity across a discrete subaortic stenosis will be increased post premature ventricular contraction.

10. True or False: According to the interval-strength relationship, the strength of ventricular contraction may be increased in a patient with sinus bradycardia.

BOARD REVIEW QUESTIONS - Section 4B

1. The time between each heart beat is called:
   a. interval
   b. strength
   c. systole
   d. diastole

2. In general, as the interval between each heart beat increases the strength of ventricular contraction:
   a. increases
   b. decreases
   c. varies
   d. cannot be predicted

3. The systolic contraction following a premature ventricular contraction with a compensatory pause will be:
   a. increased
   b. decreased
   c. unchanged
   d. cannot be predicted

4. The phenonmenon where there is an increase in systolic contraction following a premature ventricular contraction with a compensatory pause is called:
   a. pressure half time
   b. interval-strength
   c. systole
   d. diastole

5. According to the interval-strength relationship, the peak velocity and peak pressure gradient post premature ventricular contraction with a compensatory pause will be:
   a. increased
   b. decreased
   c. unchanged
   d. cannot be predicted

6. According to the interval-strength relationship, the strength of ventricular contraction in a patient with sinus bradycardia will be:
   a. increased
   b. decreased
   c. unchanged
   d. cannot be predicted

ANSWERS - Section 4B

Review practice answers

1. interval
2. strength
3. True
4. compensatory
5. True
6. potentiation
7. True
8. True
9. True
10. True

Board review answers

1. a
2. a
3. a
4. b
5. a
6. a

4. VALVE OPENING AND CLOSURE

The heart valves open and close due to changes in intracardiac pressures.

Mitral Valve

The mitral valve closes when left ventricular pressure exceeds left atrial pressure with the onset of ventricular systole at the start of the electrocardiogram QRS complex.

The mitral valve opens when left ventricular pressure falls below left atrial pressure with the onset of ventricular diastole at the end of the electrocardiogram T wave.

Tricuspid Valve

The tricuspid valve closes when right ventricular pressure exceeds right atrial pressure at the onset of ventricular systole at the start of the electrocardiogram QRS complex.

The tricuspid valve opens when right ventricular pressure falls below right atrial pressure at the onset of ventricular diastole at the end of the electrocardiogram T wave.

Comparing the Mitral Valve and Tricuspid Valve

The mitral valve closes before the tricuspid valve because left ventricular pressure increases at a faster rate when compared to the right ventricle during early ventricular systole.

The tricuspid valve opens before the mitral valve because right atrial pressure exceeds right ventricular pressure before the left atrium is able to overcome the left ventricular pressure.

Aortic Valve

The aortic valve opens when left ventricular systolic pressure exceeds aortic pressure in early ventricular systole. The aortic valve closes when left ventricular systolic pressure falls below aortic pressure.

Pulmonic Valve

The pulmonary valve opens when right ventricular pressure exceeds pulmonary artery pressure in early ventricular systole.

The pulmonary valve closes when right ventricular systolic pressure falls below pulmonary artery systolic pressure.

Comparing the Aortic Valve and Pulmonic Valves

The pulmonary valve opens before the aortic valve because it takes a shorter amount of time for right ventricular systolic pressure to exceed pulmonary artery pressure as compared to the time it takes the left ventricle to exceed the aortic pressure.

The pulmonary valve closes after the aortic valve because right ventricular ejection time is normally longer than left ventricular ejection time.

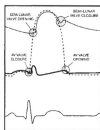

CHAPTER 4 (UNIT FOUR) - CARDIAC PHYSIOLOGY

REVIEW PRACTICE - Section 4B

1. The heart valves open and close due to a change in pressure?/volume?

2. The mitral valve opens?/closes? when left ventricular pressure exceeds left atrial pressure at the onset of ventricular systole.

3. The mitral valve opens?/closes? when left ventricular pressure falls below left atrial presssure at the onset of ventricular diastole.

4. The tricuspid valve opens?/closes? when right ventricular pressure exceeds right atrial pressure at the onset of ventricular systole.

5. The tricuspid valve opens?/closes? when right atrial pressure exceeds right ventricular pressure at the onset of ventricular diastole.

6. True or False: The tricuspid valve opens before the mitral valve.

7. True or False: The mitral valve closes before the tricuspid valve.

8. True or False: As compared to the mitral valve, the tricuspid valve opens first and closes last.

9. The aortic valve opens?/closes? when left ventricular pressure exceeds aortic pressure in early ventricular systole.

10. The aortic valve opens?/closes? when left ventricular pressure falls below aortic pressure.

11. The pulmonary valve opens?/closes? when right ventricular pressure overcomes pulmonary artery pressure in early ventricular systole.

12. The pulmonary valve opens?/closes? when right ventricular pressure falls below pulmonary artery pressure.

13. Which semilunar valve opens first: pulmonic?/aortic?

14. Which semilunar valve closes first: pulmonic?/aortic?

BOARD REVIEW QUESTIONS - Section 4B

1. The heart valves open and close due to a change in:
   a. pressure
   b. volume
   c. blood motion
   d. heart motion

2. The mitral valve closes when:
   a. left atrial pressure exceeds left ventricular pressure
   b. left ventricular systolic pressure exceeds left atrial pressure
   c. left ventricular systolic pressure exceeds aortic pressure
   d. aortic diastolic pressure exceeds left ventricular diastolic pressure

3. The mitral valve opens when:
   a. left atrial pressure exceeds left ventricular pressure
   b. left ventricular diastolic pressure exceeds left atrial pressure
   c. left ventricular systolic pressure exceeds aortic systolic pressure
   d. aortic systolic pressure exceeds left ventricularsystolic pressure

4. The tricuspid valve closes when:
   a. right atrial pressure exceeds right ventricular pressure
   b. right ventricular systolic pressure exceeds right atrial pressure
   c. right ventricular diastolic pressure exceeds pulmonary artery diastolic pressure
   d. systolic pulmonary artery pressure exceeds right ventricular systolic pressure

5. The tricuspid valve opens when:
   a. right atrial pressure exceeds right ventricular pressure
   b. right ventricular diastolic pressure exceeds right atrial pressure
   c. right ventricular systolic pressure exceeds pulmonary artery pressure
   d. systolic pulmonary artery pressure exceeds right ventricular systolic pressure

6. As compared to the mitral valve, the tricuspid valve normally opens:
   a. before
   b. at the same time
   c. after
   d. varies

7. As compared to the mitral valve, the tricuspid valve normally closes:
   a. before
   b. at the same time
   c. after
   d. varies

8. The aortic valve opens when:
    a. left atrial pressure exceeds left ventricular pressure
    b. left ventricular systolic pressure exceeds left atrial pressure
    c. left ventricular systolic pressure exceeds aortic pressure
    d. aortic systolic pressure exceeds left ventricular systolic pressure

9. The aortic valve closes when:
    a. left atrial pressure exceeds left ventricular systolic pressure
    b. left ventricular systolic pressure exceeds left atrial pressure
    c. left ventricular systolic pressure exceeds aortic diastolic pressure
    d. aortic pressure exceeds left ventricular systolic pressure

10. The pulmonary valve opens when:
    a. right atrial pressure exceeds right ventricular pressure
    b. right ventricular pressure exceeds right atrial pressure
    c. right ventricular systolic pressure exceeds pulmonary artery pressure
    d. pulmonary artery systolic pressure exceeds right ventricular pressure

11. The pulmonary valve closes when:
    a. right atrial pressure exceeds right ventricular pressure
    b. right ventricular pressure exceeds right atrial pressure
    c. right ventricular systolic pressure exceeds systolic pulmonary artery pressure
    d. systolic pulmonary artery pressure exceeds systolic right ventricular pressure

12. As compared to the aortic valve, the pulmonary valve normally opens:
    a. before
    b. at the same time
    c. after
    d. varies

13. As compared to the aortic valve, the pulmonary valve normally closes:
    a. before
    b. at the same time
    c. after
    d. varies

CHAPTER 4 (UNIT FOUR) - CARDIAC PHYSIOLOGY

ANSWERS - Section 4B

Review practice answers

1. pressure
2. closes
3. opens
4. closes
5. opens
6. True
7. True
8. True
9. opens
10. closes
11. opens
12. closes
13. pulmonic
14. aortic

Board review answers

1. a
2. b
3. a
4. b
5. a
6. a
7. c
8. c
9. d
10. c
11. d
12. a
13. c

SECTION 4C
Phases of the Cardiac Cycle
(Electro-mechanical Events)

1. VENTRICULAR DIASTOLE

Ventricular diastole is the period of the time the ventricles are filling with blood. On the electrocardiogram, ventricular diastole begins with the end of the T wave and ends with the onset of the QRS complex. During ventricular diastole, the atrioventricular valves are open, the semilunar valves are closed. The three components of ventricular diastole are rapid, early diastolic filling, diastasis (reduced diastolic filling) and atrial systole (late diastolic filling). Normally, 70% of ventricular filling occurs during the rapid, early diastolic filling phase.

2. ATRIAL SYSTOLE

Atrial systole occurs at the end of ventricular diastole with the onset of the P wave of the electrocardiogram. The atrioventricular valves are open, the semilunar valves are closed. Atrial systole normally contributes 30% to ventricular filling.

3. ISOVOLUMIC CONTRACTION

Isovolumic contraction represents the time period between atrioventricular valve closure and semilunar valve opening. All cardiac valves are closed as the ventricles begin to contract. There is an increase in ventricular pressure with no change in ventricular volume.

4. VENTRICULAR SYSTOLE

Ventricular systole represents ventricular contraction and begins with the onset of the QRS complex and ends with the T wave. The atrioventricular valves are closed and the semilunar valves are open as the ventricles eject blood into the great arteries. The two phases of ventricular systole are rapid and reduced. Ventricular volume is lowest at peak ventricular systole.

5. ISOVOLUMIC RELAXATION

Isovolumic relaxation represents the time period between semilunar valve closure and atrioventricular valve opening. This time period represents early ventricular relaxation as ventricular pressures drop with no change in ventricular volume.

REVIEW PRACTICE - Section 4C

1. Ventricular _____ begins with the end of the T wave and ends with the onset of the QRS complex.

2. During ventricular _____ the ventricles are filling with blood.

3. During ventricular diastole the atrioventricular valves are open?/closed? and the semilunar valves are open?/closed?

4. The three components of ventricular diastole are 1._____, _____ diastolic filling, 2._____ and 3._____ systole.

5. _____ is the period of time during ventricular diastole where the pressure between the atria and ventricles equilibrate.

6. True or False: Atrial systole occurs during ventricular systole.

7. Atrial systole begins with the onset of the electrocardiogram _____ wave.

8. Normally, _____% of diastolic filling occurs with atrial systole.

9. Normally, _____% of diastolic filling occurs with rapid, early diastolic filling.

10. _____ contraction occurs between atroventricular valve closure and semilunar valve opening.

11. True or False: During isovolumic contraction, there is an increase in ventricular volume with no change in ventricular pressure.

12. Ventricular _____ represents ventricular contraction beginning at the onset of the electrocardiogram QRS complex to the end of the T wave.

13. During ventricular systole, the atrioventricular valves are open?/closed? and the semilunar valves are open?/closed?

14. _____relaxation represents the time period from semilunar valve closure to atrioventricular valve opening.

15. True or False: During isovolumic relaxation, the ventricular pressures increase while the ventricular volumes remain unchanged.

BOARD REVIEW QUESTIONS - Section 4C

1. Which of the following begins with the end of the electrocardiogram T wave and ends with the onset of the QRS complex?
    a. ventricular diastole
    b. atrial systole
    c. ventricular systole
    d. isovolumic relaxation

2. Which of the following are true statements concerning the cardiac valves during ventricular diastole?
    a. atrioventricular valves are open, semilunar valves are closed
    b. atrioventricular valves are closed, semilunar valves are open
    c. atrioventricular valves are open, semilunar valves are open
    d. atrioventricular valves are closed, semilunar valves are closed

3. All of the following are considered components of ventricular diastole except:
    a. rapid early filling
    b. diastasis
    c. atrial systole
    d. isovolumic contraction

4. Atrial systole is considered a part of:
    a. early diastolic filling
    b. diastasis
    c. mid-ventricular diastole
    d. late ventricular diastole

5. What percentage does atrial systole normally contribute to ventricular diastolic filling?
    a. 10%
    b. 30%
    c. 70%
    d. 90%

6. What percentage does rapid, early diastolic filling contribute to ventricular diastolic filling?
    a. 10%
    b. 30%
    c. 70%
    d. 90%

7. The period of time between atrioventricular valve closure and semilunar valve opening is called:
   a. rapid, early diastolic filling
   b. diastasis
   c. atrial systole
   d. isovolumic contraction

8. Which of the following statements is true concerning isovolumic contraction?
   a. atrioventricular valves are open, semilunar valves are closed
   b. atrioventricular valves are closed, semilunar valves are open
   c. atrioventricular valves are open, semilunar valves are open
   d. atrioventricular valves are closed, semilunar valves are closed

9. During isovolumic contraction, the ventricular pressure is _____ and the ventricular volume is _____.
   a. increased, decreased
   b. increased, increased
   c. increased, no change
   d. varies, varies

10. Which component of the electrocardiogram tracing represents ventricular systole?
    a. P wave
    b. QRS complex to T wave
    c. T wave to QRS complex
    d. T wave to onset of P wave

11. Which of the following statements is true concerning the cardiac valves during ventricular systole?
    a. atrioventricular valves are open, semilunar valves are closed
    b. atrioventricular valves are closed, semilunar valves are open
    c. atrioventricular valves are open, semilunar valves are open
    d. atrioventricular valves are closed, semilunar valves are closed

12. The period of time between semilunar valve closure and atrioventricular valve opening is:
    a. atrial systole
    b. ventricular diastole
    c. ventricular diastasis
    d. isovolumic relaxation

13. Which of the following statements is true concerning isovolumic relaxation?
    a. ventricular pressure and volume are increasing
    b. ventricular pressure and volume are decreasing
    c. ventricular pressure is increasing, ventricular volume is unchanged
    d. ventricular pressure is decreasing, ventricular volume is unchanged

ANSWERS - Section 4C

Review practice answers

1. diastole
2. diastole
3. open, closed
4. rapid early, diastasis, atrial
5. diastasis
6. False
7. P
8. 30
9. 70
10. isovolumic
11. False
12. systole
13. closed, open
14. isovolumic
15. False

Board review answers

1. a
2. a
3. d
4. d
5. b
6. c
7. d
8. d
9. c
10. b
11. b
12. d
13. d

SECTION 4D
Left Ventricular Function: Indicators and Normal Values

1. STROKE VOLUME (SV)

Stroke volume is the amount of blood pumped out of the heart per beat.

Formula: End-diastolic volume (EDV) - end-systolic volume (ESV)

Units: cubic centimeters (cc) or milliliters (ml)

Normal range: 70 cc to 100 cc

M-mode, two dimensional and cardiac Doppler echocardiography may be used to calculate stroke volume. The cardiac Doppler formula for stroke volume is: CSA x VTI where CSA represents the cross-sectional area and VTI is the velocity time integral.

2. EJECTION FRACTION (EF)

Ejection fraction is the percentage of blood pumped out of the heart per beat.

Formula: $\underline{\text{End-diastolic volume (EDV) - end-systolic volume (ESV)}}$ x 100

                         End-diastolic volume (EDV)

Units: Expressed as a percentage

Normal range: $62 \pm 12\%$

M-mode and two dimensional echocardiography may be used to calculate ejection fraction.

3. CARDIAC OUTPUT (CO)

Cardiac output is the amount of blood pumped out of the heart per minute.

Formula: Stroke volume (SV) x heart rate (HR)

Units: liters per minute (lpm)

Normal range: 4 lpm to 8 lpm

M-mode, two-D and cardiac Doppler echocardiography may be used to calculate cardiac output.

4. CARDIAC INDEX (CI)

Cardiac index is the cardiac output adjusted for body surface area.

Formula: Cardiac output (CO)/body surface area (BSA)

Units: lpm/m^2

Normal range: $2.4 \ lpm/m^2$ to $4.2 \ lpm/m^2$

M-mode, two dimensional and cardiac Doppler echocardiography may be used to calculate cardiac index.

REVIEW PRACTICE - Section 4D

1.   The amount of blood pumped out of the heart per beat is called: _____ _____.

2.   The formula for stroke volume is: _____ _____ volume - _____ _____ volume.

3.   The units for stroke volume are _____ _____ (___) or _____ (___).

4.   The normal range for stroke volume is _____ cc to _____ cc.

5.   True False: The only echo-Doppler technique that may be used to calculate stroke volume is cardiac Doppler.

6.   The left ventricular outflow tract diameter measures 2.0 cm and the velocity time integral is 20 cm. The stroke volume by cardiac Doppler is:_____ cc.

7.   The amount of blood pumped out of the heart per minute is called _____ _____.

8.   The formula for cardiac output is _____ _____ x _____ _____.

9.   The units for cardiac output are _____ per _____.

10. The normal range for cardiac output is _____ lpm to _____ lpm.

11. Cardiac output adjusted for body surface area is _____ _____.

12. The formula for cardiac index is _____ _____/_____ surface area.

13. The units for cardiac index are liters per minute /_____ squared.

14. The normal range for cardiac index is _____ lpm/m^2 to _____ lpm/m^2.

15. The percentage of blood pumped from the heart per beat is called _____ _____

16. The formula for ejection fraction is _____ _____ volume - _____ _____ volume /_____ _____ volume x 100.

17. True or False: Ejection fraction = stroke volume/end-diastolic volume x 100.

18. True or False: Ejection fraction may be expressed as a percentage.

19. The normal range for ejection fraction is _____ $\pm$ 12%.

20. True or False: M-mode, two-dimensional and cardiac Doppler may all be used to calculate ejection fraction.

BOARD REVIEW QUESTIONS - Section 4D

1. The amount of blood pumped out of the heart per beat is:
    a. stroke volume
    b. cardiac output
    c. cardiac index
    d. ejection fraction

2. The formula for stroke volume is:
    a. end-diastolic volume - end-systolic volume
    b. end-diastolic volume - end-systolic volume x heart rate
    c. cardiac output/body surface area
    d. end-diastolic volume - end-systolic volume/end-diastolic volume

3. The units for stroke volume are:
    a. cubic centimeters
    b. liters per minute
    c. liters per minute/meter squared
    d. percentage

4. The normal range for stroke volume is:
    a. 70 cc to 100 cc
    b. 4 lpm to 8 lpm
    c. 2.4 lpm/m^2 to 4.2 lpm/m^2
    d. 62% $\pm$ 12%

5. Stroke volume may be calculated by each of the following modalities except:
    a. A-mode
    b. M-mode
    c. two-dimensional
    d. cardiac Doppler

6. The amount of blood pumped out of the heart per minute is:
    a. stroke volume
    b. cardiac output
    c. cardiac index
    d. ejection fraction

7. The formula for cardiac output is:
    a. end-diastolic volume - end-systolic volume
    b. end-diastolic volume - end-systolic volume x heart rate
    c. stroke volume x heart rate/body surface area
    d. stroke volume/end-diastolic volume x 100

8. The units for cardiac output are:
    a. cubic centimeters
    b. liters per minute
    c. liters per minute/body surface area
    d. percentage

9. The normal range for cardiac output is:
    a. 70 cc to 100 cc
    b. 4 lpm to 8 lpm
    c. 2.4 lpm/m^2 to 4.2 lpm/m^2
    d. 62 % $\pm$ 12%

10. Cardiac output may be calculated by all of the following modalities except:
    a. A-mode
    b. M-mode
    c. two-dimensional
    d. cardiac Doppler

11. Cardiac output adjusted for body surface area is:
    a. stroke volume
    b. body surface area
    c. cardiac index
    d. ejection fraction

12. The formula for cardiac index is:
    a. end-diastolic volume - end-systolic volume
    b. end-diastolic volume - end-systolic volume x heart rate
    c. stroke volume x heart rate/body surface area
    d. stroke volume/end-diastolic volume

13. The units for cardiac index are:
    a. cubic centimeters
    b. liters per minute
    c. liters per minute/meter squared
    d. percentage

14. The normal range for cardiac index is:
    a. 70 cc to 100 cc
    b. 4 lpm to 8 lpm
    c. 2.4 lpm/m^2 to 4.2 lpm/m^2
    d. 62% $\pm$ 12%

15. All of the following modalities may calculate cardiac index except:
    a. A-mode
    b. M-mode
    c. two-dimensional
    d. cardiac Doppler

16. The percentage of blood pumped out of the heart per beat is:
    a. stroke volume
    b. cardiac output
    c. cardiac index
    d. ejection fraction

17. The formula for ejection fraction is:
    a. end-diastolic volume - end-systolic volume
    b. stroke volume x heart rate
    c. stroke volume x heart rate/body surface area
    d. stroke volume/end-diastolic volume x 100

18. Ejection fraction may be expressed as:
    a. cubic centimeters
    b. liters per minute
    c. liters per minute/meter squared
    d. a percentage

19. The normal range for ejection fraction is:
    a. 70 cc to 100 cc
    b. 4 lpm to 8 lpm
    c. 2.4 lpm/m^2 to 4.2 lpm/m^2
    d. 62% $\pm$ 12%

20. All of the following modalities may calculate ejection fraction except:
    a. M-mode
    b. two-dimensional
    c. cardiac Doppler
    d. multigated equilibrium study

21. The left ventricular outflow tract measures 2.0 cm. The time velocity integral is 15 cm. The cardiac Doppler stroke volume is equal to:
    a. 2.0 cm
    b. 15 cm
    c. 30 cc
    d. 47 cc

ANSWERS - Section 4D

Review practice answers

1. stroke volume
2. end-diastolic, end-systolic
3. cubic centimeters (cc), milliliters (ml)
4. 70, 100
5. False
6. 62.8 cc
7. cardiac output
8. stroke volume, heart rate
9. liters, minute
10. 4, 8
11. cardiac index
12. cardiac output, body
13. meters
14. 2.4, 4.2
15. ejection fraction
16. end-diastolic, end-systolic, end-diastolic
17. True
18. True
19. 62
20. False

Board review answers

1.	a	18.	d
2.	a	19.	d
3.	a	20.	c
4.	a	21.	d
5.	a		
6.	b		
7.	b		
8.	b		
9.	b		
10.	a		
11.	c		
12.	c		
13.	c		
14.	c		
15.	a		
16.	d		
17.	d		

SECTION 4E
Pulmonary vs Systemic Circulation

Components of the Pulmonary Circulation

The following are considered a component of the pulmonary circulation:
> right ventricle
> main pulmonary artery and branches
> pulmonary capillaries
> pulmonary veins

Components of the Systemic Circulation

The following are considered a component of the systemic circulation:
> left ventricle
> aorta
> systemic capillary network
> cerebral, peripheral and abdominal veins
> superior vena cava and inferior vena cava

Comparing the Systemic Circulation and Pulmonary Circulation

When comparing the systemic circulation to the pulmonary circulation the systemic circulation has:
> higher pressure
> higher resistance
> higher O2 content
> lower carbon dioxide content
> thicker ventricular walls
> higher overall volume
> thicker vessel walls
> blood traveling a greater distance
> equal stroke volume

REVIEW PRACTICE - Section 4E

1. Check the following if considered a component of the pulmonary circulation:

    _____right ventricle

    _____main pulmonary artery and branches

    _____pulmonary capillaries

    _____pulmonary veins

2. Check the following if considered a component of the systemic circulation:

    _____left ventricle

    _____aorta

    _____systemic capillary network

    _____cerebral, peripheral, abdominal veins

    _____superior vena cava and inferior vena cava

Tell if the following statements are True or False when comparing the systemic circulation to the pulmonary circulation:

3. _____The systemic circulation is a higher pressure system than the pulmonary circulation.

4. _____The systemic circulation is a higher resistance system than the pulmonary circulation.

5. _____The systemic circulation has a lower oxygen content than the pulmonary circulation.

6. _____The systemic circulation has a lower carbon dioxide content.

7. _____The left ventricular walls are thicker than the right ventricular walls.

8. _____The systemic circulation contains a higher volume of blood than does the pulmonary circulation.

9. _____The systemic vessel walls are thicker than the pulmonary system vessel walls.

10. _____The systemic circulation has blood traveling a greater distance than the pulmonary circulation.

11. _____The left ventricular stroke volume is greater than the right ventricular stroke volume.

BOARD REVIEW QUESTIONS - Section 4E

1. All of the following are considered a part of the pulmonary circulation except:
   a. vena cava
   b. right ventricle
   c. pulmonary artery and branches
   d. pulmonary capillaries

2. All of the following are considered components of the systemic circulation except:
   a. pulmonary veins
   b. left ventricle
   c. aorta
   d. cerebral veins

3. All of the following are true statements comparing the systemic circulation to the pulmonary circulation except:
   a. higher pressure
   b. higher resistance
   c. higher O2 content
   d. higher carbon dioxide content

4. All of the following are true statements comparing the systemic circulation to the pulmonary circulation except:
   a. higher overall volume
   b. thicker vessel walls
   c. blood travels a greater distance
   d. higher stroke volume

5. The left ventricular stroke volume as compared to the right ventricular stroke volume is:
   a. 10% greater
   b. 10% less
   c. equal to
   d. cannot be predicted

ANSWERS - Section 4E

Review practice answers

1. all
2. all
3. True
4. True
5. False
6. True
7. True
8. True
9. True
10. True
11. False

Board review answers

1. a
2. a
3. d
4. d
5. c

Intracardiac Pressures and Principles of Flow

1. NORMAL VALUES (mm Hg)

Systemic arterial
peak systolic/end diastolic	100 to 140/60 to 90
mean	70 to 105
systolic mean	80 to 130

Left ventricle
peak systolic/end diastolic	100 to 140/3 to 12
systolic mean/diastolic mean	80 to 130/1 to 10

Left atrium or pulmonary wedge
mean	2 to 12
a wave	3 to 15
v wave	3 to 15
diastolic mean	1 to 10

Pulmonary artery
peak systolic/end diastolic	15 to 30/4 to 12
mean	9 to 18
systolic mean	10 to 20

Right ventricle
peak systolic/end diastolic	15 to 30/2 to 8
systolic mean/diastolic mean	10 to 20/0 to 4

Right atrium
mean	2 to 8
a wave	2 to 10
v wave	2 to 10

INTRACARDIAC PRESSURES

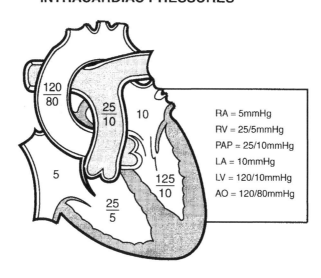

RA = 5mmHg
RV = 25/5mmHg
PAP = 25/10mmHg
LA = 10mmHg
LV = 120/10mmHg
AO = 120/80mmHg

CHAPTER 4 (UNIT FOUR) - CARDIAC PHYSIOLOGY

REVIEW PRACTICE - Section 4F

1. The normal range for systemic arterial peak systolic pressure is: _____mm Hg to _____ mm Hg.

2. The normal range for the systemic arterial end diastolic pressure is:_____mm Hg to _____mm Hg.

3. The normal range for the mean systemic arterial pressure is:_____ mm Hg to _____ mm Hg.

4. The normal peak systolic left ventricular pressure range is:_____ mm Hg to _____ mm Hg.

5. The normal range for left ventricular end diastolic pressure is:_____ mm Hg to _____ mm Hg.

6. The normal range for the mean left atrial or pulmonary wedge pressure is:_____ mm Hg to _____ mm Hg.

7. The normal range for the a wave of the left atrium or pulmonary wedge pressure is:_____mm Hg to _____mm Hg.

8. The normal pressure range for the v wave of the left atrium or pulmonary wedge pressure is:_____ mm Hg to _____ mm Hg.

9. The normal range for the pulmonary artery systolic pressure is:_____ mm Hg to _____ mm Hg.

10. The normal range for the pulmonary artery end diastolic pressure is: _____ mm Hg to _____ mm Hg.

11. The normal range for the mean pulmonary artery pressure is _____ mm Hg to _____ mm Hg.

12. The normal range for the peak systolic right ventricular pressure is: _____mm Hg to _____ mm Hg.

13. The normal range for the right ventricular end diastolic pressure is: _____ mm Hg to _____ mm Hg.

14. The normal range for the right atrial mean pressure is: _____ mm Hg to _____ mm Hg.

15. The normal range for the right atrial a wave pressure is: _____ mm Hg to _____ mm Hg.

16. The normal range for the right atrial v wave pressure is: _____ mm Hg to _____ mm Hg.

17. In the absence of right ventricular inflow tract obstruction, the right atrial pressure reflects the right ventricular _____ pressure.

18. In the absence of right ventricular outflow tract obstruction, the right ventricular systolic pressure equals the pulmonary artery _____ pressure.

19. The pulmonary artery end diastolic pressure equals the left _____ and left ventricular _____ pressure.

20. In the absence of left ventricular outflow tract obstruction, the systolic blood pressure equals the left ventricular _____ pressure.

BOARD REVIEW QUESTIONS - Section 4F

1. Which of the following best represents the normal range for systemic arterial peak systolic pressure?
    a. 70 mm Hg to 105 mm Hg
    b. 3 mm Hg to 12 mm Hg
    c. 15 mm Hg to 30 mm Hg
    d. 100 mm Hg to 140 mm Hg

2. Which of the following best represents the normal mean systemic arterial pressure range?
    a. 100 mm Hg to 140 mm Hg
    b. 15 mm Hg to 30 mm Hg
    c. 3 mm Hg to 12 mm Hg
    d. 60 mm Hg to 90 mm Hg

3. Which of the following best represents the normal systemic arterial end diastolic pressure range?
    a. 100 mm Hg to 140 mm Hg
    b. 15 mm Hg to 30 mm Hg
    c. 2 mm Hg to 10 mm Hg
    d. 60 mm Hg to 90 mm Hg

4. Which of the following best represents the normal left ventricular end diastolic pressure range?
    a. 3 mm Hg to 12 mm Hg
    b. 15 mm Hg to 30 mm Hg
    c. 80 mm Hg to 130 mm Hg
    d. 100 mm Hg to 140 mm Hg

5. The normal range for mean left atrial/pulmonary wedge pressure is:
    a. 2 mm Hg to 12 mm Hg
    b. 60 mm Hg to 90 mm Hg
    c. 70 mm Hg to 105 mm Hg
    d. 100 mm Hg to 140 mm Hg

6. The normal range for pulmonary artery peak systolic pressure is:
    a. 4 mm Hg to 12 mm Hg
    b. 15 mm Hg to 30 mm Hg
    c. 80 mm Hg to 130 mm Hg
    d. 100 mm Hg to 140 mm Hg

7. The normal range for pulmonary artery end-diastolic pressure is:
    a. 3 mm Hg to 15 mm Hg
    b. 9 mm Hg to 18 mm Hg
    c. 4 mm Hg to 12 mm Hg
    d. 100 mm Hg to 140 mm Hg

8. The normal range for the mean pulmonary artery pressure is:
    a. 2 mm Hg to 12 mm Hg
    b. 9 mm Hg to 18 mm Hg
    c. 15 mm Hg to 30 mmHg
    d. 70 mm Hg to 105 mm Hg

9. The normal range for the right ventricular peak systolic pressure is:
    a. 2 mm Hg to 8 mm Hg
    b. 15 mm Hg to 30 mm Hg
    c. 80 mm Hg to 130 mm Hg
    d. 100 mm Hg to 140 mm Hg

10. The normal range for the right ventricular end diastolic pressure is:
    a. 2 mm Hg to 8 mm Hg
    b. 15 mm Hg to 30 mm Hg
    c. 70 mm Hg to 105 mm Hg
    d. 100 mm Hg to 140 mm Hg

11. The normal range for the mean right atrial pressure is:
    a. 2 mm Hg to 8 mm Hg
    b. 15 mm Hg to 30 mm Hg
    c. 60 mm Hg to 90 mm Hg
    d. 100 mm Hg to 140 mm Hg

12. Normally the peak arterial systolic pressure is equal to the peak systolic:
    a. right atrium
    b. right ventricle
    c. pulmonary artery
    d. left ventricle

13. Normally the left ventricular diastolic pressure is equal to the diastolic pressure of the:
    a. right atrium
    b. left atrium
    c. right ventricle
    d. left ventricle

CHAPTER 4 (UNIT FOUR) - CARDIAC PHYSIOLOGY

14. The left atrial/pulmonary artery wedge pressure normally represents the diastolic pressure of the:
    a. right atrium
    b. right ventricle
    c. pulmonary artery
    d. left ventricle

15. The peak right ventricular systolic pressure normally is equal to the:
    a. right atrium
    b. pulmonary artery peak systolic
    c. left atrium
    d. left ventricular peak systolic

16. The mean right atrial pressure normally is equal to the:
    a. left atrium
    b. left ventricle end diastolic
    c. mean pulmonary artery
    d. right ventricular diastolic

ANSWERS - Section 4F

Review practice answers

1. 100, 140
2. 60, 90
3. 70, 105
4. 100, 140
5. 3, 12
6. 2, 12
7. 3, 15
8. 3, 15
9. 15, 30
10. 4, 12
11. 9, 18
12. 15, 30
13. 2, 8
14. 2, 8
15. 2, 10
16. 2, 10
17. diastolic
18. systolic
19. atrial, diastolic
20. systolic

Board review answers

1. d
2. d
3. d
4. a
5. a
6. b
7. c
8. b
9. b
10. a
11. a
12. d
13. b
14. d
15. b
16. d

2. CHANGES DURING THE CARDIAC CYCLE

Blood flows from a higher pressure chamber to a lower pressure chamber.

A change in pressure causes cardiac valves to open and close.

There will be an increase in the pressure of a chamber located proximal to an obstruction and a decrease in the pressure of the chamber distal to the obstruction, i.e. left ventricular systolic pressure will increase in valvular aortic stenosis while the systolic aortic pressure will be decreased.

The following pressure changes due to the following abnormalities should be noted:

Mitral regurgitation and tricuspid regurgitation may cause large atrial v waves and/or the merging of the atrial c and v waves.

Mitral stenosis and tricuspid stenosis may cause an increase in atrial a waves, although atrial a waves will be absent in patients with atrial fibrillation.

Constrictive pericarditis is associated with steep x and y descents of the atrial pressure tracing.

Systemic hypertension, pulmonary hypertension and/or semilunar valve obstruction will increase ventricular systolic pressure.

Congestive heart failure, constrictive pericarditis and diastolic dysfunction may increase ventricular end diastolic pressure.

Left to right shunts (e.g. atrial septal defect, ventricular septal defect, patent ductus arteriosus) or left heart disease may increase pulmonary artery pressures.

REVIEW PRACTICE - Section 4F

1. True or False: Blood flows from a higher pressure chamber to a lower pressure chamber.

2. True or False: A change in pressure causes cardiac valves to open and close.

3. True or False: There will be an increase in pressure in the chamber distal to an obstruction.

4. Mitral regurgitation and tricuspid regurgitation may cause the atrial ___ wave to be increased.

5. True or False: There will be no atrial a wave in patients with atrial fibrillation.

6. Mitral and tricuspid stenosis will cause the atrial _____ wave to be increased.

7. _____ pericarditis is associated with steep x and y descents.

8. True or False: Hypertension will increase ventricular systolic pressure.

9. True or False: Semi-lunar valve stenosis will decrease ventricular systolic pressure.

10. True or False: Congestive heart failure may lead to an increase in left ventricular end diastolic pressure.

11. True or False: Constrictive pericarditis may lead to an increase in left ventricular end diastolic pressure.

12. True or False: Left ventricular diastolic dysfunction may lead to an increase in left ventricular end diastolic pressure.

13. True or False: A left to right shunt may decrease pulmonary artery pressures.

14. True or False: Pulmonary hypertension implies an increase in pulmonary artery pressures.

15. True or False: Left heart disease may lead to an increase in left ventricular end diastolic pressures, left atrial pressures, and pulmonary artery pressures.

BOARD REVIEW QUESTIONS - Section 4F

1. Assuming normal intracardiac pressures, all of the following statements are true concerning blood flow during ventricular systole except blood travels from the:
    a.   left ventricle to the aorta
    b.   right ventricle to the pulmonary artery
    c.   vena cava to the right atrium
    d.   left atrium to the pulmonary veins

2. When early ventricular systolic pressure exceeds atrial pressures the atrioventricular valves will:
    a.   open
    b.   close
    c.   be unaffected
    d.   cannot be predicted

3. When ventricular systolic pressure exceeds arterial pressure the semi-lunar valves will:
    a.   open
    b.   close
    c.   be unaffected
    d.   cannot be predicted

4. When ventricular diastolic pressure falls below arterial pressure the semi-lunar valves will:
    a.   open
    b.   close
    c.   be unaffected
    d.   cannot be predicted

5. When ventricular pressure falls below atrial pressure the atrioventricular valves will:
    a.   open
    b.   close
    c.   be unaffected
    d.   cannot be predicted

6. Atrioventricular valve regurgitation will increase the atrial wave called the:
    a.   a
    b.   c
    c.   x
    d.   v

7. Atrial fibrillation will cause which of the following atrial waves to be absent?
   a. a
   b. c
   c. x
   d. v

8. Atrioventricular valve stenosis will lead to an increase in the atrial wave called the:
   a. a wave
   b. c wave
   c. x wave
   d. v wave

9. Which of the following cardiac diseases is associated with steep atrial x and y descents?
   a. mitral regurgitation
   b. tricuspid stenosis
   c. constrictive pericarditis
   d. semilunar valve stenosis

10. All of the following will directly increase ventricular systolic pressure except:
   a. aortic stenosis
   b. mitral stenosis
   c. systemic hypertension
   d. pulmonary hypertension

11. All of the following cardiac diseases will lead to an increase in left ventricular end diastolic pressure except:
   a. congestive heart failure
   b. constrictive pericarditis
   c. tricuspid stenosis
   d. diastolic dysfunction

12. All of the following may increase pulmonary artery pressures except:
   a. atrial septal defect
   b. coronary artery disease
   c. mitrial stenosis
   d. tricuspid regurgitation

ANSWERS - Section 4F

Review practice answers

1. True
2. True
3. False
4. v
5. True
6. a
7. constrictive
8. True
9. False
10. True
11. True
12. True
13. False
14. True
15. True

Board review answers

1. d
2. b
3. a
4. b
5. a
6. d
7. a
8. a
9. c
10. b
11. c
12. d

3. OXYGEN SATURATION

The vena cava, right atrium, right ventricle and main pulmonary artery have an oxygen saturation value of approximately 75%. The superior vena cava has a slightly lower oxygen saturation because it receives the desaturated blood from the brain. The coronary sinus has an oxygen saturation of 60%, which is the lowest level in the body.

The pulmonary veins, left atrium, left ventricle and aorta have an oxygen saturation of 98%.

INTRACARDIAC 02 SATURATIONS

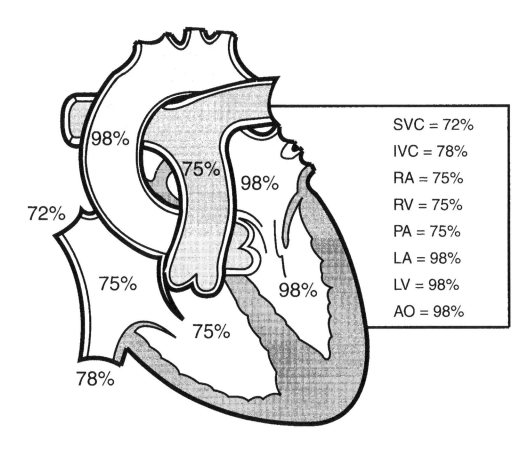

SVC = 72%
IVC = 78%
RA = 75%
RV = 75%
PA = 75%
LA = 98%
LV = 98%
AO = 98%

REVIEW PRACTICE - Section 4F

1.   The oxygen saturation for the right heart chambers is normally _____%

2.   True or False: The superior vena cava has a slightly lower oxygen saturation when compared to the rest of the right heart structures.

3.   True or False: The coronary sinus has the lowest oxygen saturation of any structure in the body.

4.   The oxygen saturation for the left heart is normally _____%.

BOARD REVIEW QUESTIONS - Section 4F

1. The right heart oxygen saturations normally are equal to approximately:
    a. 25%
    b. 50%
    c. 75%
    d. 95%

2. Which of the following will normally have the lowest oxygen saturation level?
    a. inferior vena cava
    b. superior vena cava
    c. right atrium
    d. pulmonary vein

3. The normal oxygen saturation level for the left heart is:
    a. 25%
    b. 50%
    c. 75%
    d. 95%

4. Which of the following normally has the lowest oxygen saturation level?
    a. vena cava
    b. coronary sinus
    c. pulmonary veins
    d. aorta

5. Which of the following normally has the highest oxygen saturation level?
    a. aorta
    b. left atrium
    c. left ventricle
    d. pulmonary veins

ANSWERS - Section 4F

Review practice answers

1. 75%
2. True
3. True
4. 98%

Board review answers

1. c
2. b
3. d
4. b
5. d

SECTION 4G
Maneuvers Altering Cardiac Physiology

Certain maneuvers may be utilized by the physician during cardiac auscultation to enhance or bring about cardiac murmurs. The sonographer may utilize these same maneuvers to prove the presence of cardiac pathology.

Positional Changes

Supine to standing: Standing will reduce venous return, ventricular stroke volume and cardiac output causing a reflex increase in heart rate and systemic vascular resistance. Supine to standing will reduce the intensity of all murmurs except for hypertrophic obstructive cardiomyopathy and mitral valve prolapse.

Standing to supine: Sudden recumbency will increase venous return and ventricular stroke volume. The mid-systolic ejection murmurs of valvular aortic and pulmonic stenosis will increase in intensity while the murmurs of hypertrophic obstructive cardiomyopathy and mitral valve prolapse will decrease in intensity.

Passive leg raising: Passive leg raising has the same physiologic effects as does sudden recumbency.

Standing to squatting: Prompt squatting will increase venous return and ventricular stroke volume. Squatting causes most murmurs to increase except for the murmurs of hypertrophic obstructive cardiomyopathy and mitral valve prolapse, which will decrease.

Standing to walking: Standing to walking will increase venous return, stroke volume, cardiac output and heart rate.

Maneuvers

Valsalva maneuver: The strain phase of the Valsalva maneuver results in an increase in intrathoracic pressure therefore decreasing venous return, stroke volume and cardiac output. All murmurs will decrease in intensity during the Valsalva maneuver except for the murmurs of hypertrophic obstructive cardiomyopathy and mitral valve prolapse. During the release phase there is an increase in venous return. This is useful when evaluating for patent foramen ovale (PFO) during a contrast saline study.

Isometric handgrip: The handgrip increases peripheral vascular resistance, blood pressure and heart rate. Mitral regurgitation, aortic regurgitation and ventricular septal defect murmurs will increase in intensity during isometric handgrip. The murmurs of semi-lunar valve stenosis and hypertrophic obstructive cardiomyopathy will decrease in intensity.

Pharmacological Interventions

Amyl nitrite: Amyl nitrite is a vasodilator which causes a decrease in venous return and blood pressure. The murmurs of aortic stenosis, aortic sclerosis and hypertrophic obstructive cardiomyopathy are increased. The murmur of mitral valve prolapse may be elicited. The murmurs of mitral regurgitation, aortic regurgitation and ventricular septal defect will decrease in intensity.

Respiration

Inspiration: Inspiration increases venous return and ventricular stroke volume. The murmurs of tricuspid regurgitation, pulmonary regurgitation, tricuspid stenosis and pulmonic stenosis will increase in intensity due to the increase in venous return upon inspiration. Inspiration will increase the splitting of the S2 (time interval between closure of aortic valve and pulmonic valve) as well as augment right heart S3 and S4 heart sounds.

Expiration: Expiration decreases venous return and ventricular stroke volume. All murmurs that originate from the left heart will be increased in intensity. All right heart murmurs will decrease in intensity during expiration. The splitting of S2, (time interval between aortic valve closure and pulmonic valve closure) will decrease with expiration.

ARIZONA HEART FOUNDATION

REVIEW PRACTICE - Section 4G

1. Supine to standing will increase?/decrease? venous return, ventricular stroke volume and cardiac output.

2. True or False: Supine to standing will decrease the intensity of all murmurs except the murmurs of hypertrophic obstructive cardiomyopathy and mitral valve prolapse.

3. Standing to supine will increase?/decrease? venous return and ventricular stroke volume.

4. The mid-systolic ejection murmurs of valvular aortic stenosis and pulmonic stenosis will increase?/decrease? in intensity with a change in position from standing to supine.

5. True or False: Supine to standing will decrease the intensity of the murmurs of hypertrophic obstructive cardiomyopathy and mitral valve prolapse.

6. True or False: Passive leg raising will have the same physiologic effects as standing to supine.

7. Standing to squatting will increase?/decrease? venous return and ventricular volume.

8. With standing to squatting, the murmurs of mitral regurgitation and tricuspid regurgitation will increase?/decrease? in intensity.

9. With standing to squatting, the murmurs of hypertrophic obstructive cardiomyopathy and mitral valve prolapse will increase?/decrease? in intensity.

10. The strain phase of the Valsalva maneuver will increase?/decrease? venous return and ventricular stroke volume.

11. All murmurs except hypertrophic obstructive cardiomyopathy and mitral valve prolapse will increase?/decrease? in intensity during the Valsalva maneuver.

12. True or False: The isometric handgrip will increase peripheral vascular resistance, blood pressure and heart rate.

13. The murmurs of mitral regurgitation, aortic regurgitation and ventricular septal defect will increase?/decrease? in intensity during the isometric handgrip.

14. The murmurs of valvular aortic stenosis, valvular pulmonic stenosis and hypertrophic obstructive cardiomyopathy will increase?/decrease? in intensity during the isometric handgrip.

15. Initially, the inhalation of amyl nitrite will increase?/decrease? venous return.

16. True or False: The murmurs of aortic valve stenosis, aortic sclerosis and hypertrophic obstructive cardiomyopathy increase during amyl nitrite inhalation.

17. True or False: The murmurs of ventnricular septal defect, mitral regurgitation and aortic regurgitation decrease with the inhalation of amyl nitrite.

18. True or False: Amyl nitrite inhalation may elicit or enhance mitral valve prolapse.

19. Inspiration increases?/decreases? venous return and ventricular stroke volume.

20. Inspiration increases?/decreases? the time interval between the closure of the aortic valve and pulmonic valve.

21. True or False: With inspiration most right heart murmurs and heart sounds will decrease in intensity.

22. Expiration increases?/decreases? venous return and ventricular stroke volume.

23. With expiration, all left heart murmurs will increase?/decrease? in intensity.

24. With expiration, all right heart murmurs will increase?/decrease? in intensity.

BOARD REVIEW QUESTIONS - 4G

1. What effect will supine to standing have on venous return and ventricular volume?
    a. increase
    b. no change
    c. decrease
    d. cannot be determined

2. Supine to standing will increase the intensity of all murmurs except:
    a. aortic regurgitation
    b. mitral regurgitation
    c. hypertrophic obstructive cardiomyopathy
    d. valvular aortic stenosis

3. What effect will standing to supine have on venous return and ventricular stroke volume?
    a. increase
    b. none
    c. decrease
    d. cannot be predicted

4. Standing to supine will increase the intensity of all of the following murmurs except:
    a. valvular aortic stenosis
    b. valvular pulmonic stenosis
    c. hypertrophic obstructive cardiomyopathy
    d. congenital semilunar valve stenosis

5. Which of the following has the same physiologic effect as standing to supine?
    a. inspiration
    b. isometric handgrip
    c. passive leg raising
    d. Valsalva maneuver

6. Which effect will standing to squatting have on venous return and ventricular stroke volume.
    a. increase
    b. no change
    c. decrease
    d. cannot be predicted

7. All of the following murmurs will increase in intensity with prompt squatting except:
    a. mitral regurgitation
    b. aortic regurgitation
    c. hypertrophic obstructive cardiomyopathy
    d. mitral regurgitation

8. What effect will the strain phase of the Valsalva maneuver have on venous return and ventricular stroke volume?
   a. increase
   b. no change
   c. decrease
   d. cannot be predicted

9. Which of the following murmurs will increase in intensity with the Valsalva maneuver?
   a. aortic regurgitation
   b. mitral regurgitation
   c. valvular aortic stenosis
   d. hypertrophic obstructive cardiomyopathy

10. The isometric handgrip will increase all of the following except:
    a. respirations
    b. peripheral vascular resistance
    c. blood pressure
    d. heart rate

11. Concerning the isometric handgrip, which of the following is incorrectly matched?
    a. mitral regurgitation: increased intensity
    b. aortic regurgitation: increased intensity
    c. valvular aortic stenosis: decreased intensity
    d. valvular pulmonic stenosis: increased intensity

12. The inhalation of amyl nitrite will increase all of the following murmurs except:
    a. valvular aortic stenosis
    b. valvular aortic sclerosis
    c. hypertrophic obstructive cardiomyopathy
    d. ventricular septal defect

13. Amyl nitrite inhalation may elicit or enhance:
    a. mitral valve prolapse
    b. ventricular septal defect
    c. aortic regurgitation
    d. mitral regurgitation

14. What effect will inspiration have on venous return and ventricular stroke volume?
    a. increase
    b. no change
    c. decrease
    d. cannot be predicted

15. All of the following will increase in intensity with inspiration except:
    a. tricuspid regurgitation
    b. mitral regurgitation
    c. valvular pulmonic stenosis
    d. right heart S3

16. What effect will inspiration have on the time interval between aortic valve closure and pulmonic valve closure.
    a. increase
    b. no change
    c. decrease
    d. cannot be predicted

17. What effect will expiration have on venous return and ventricular stroke volume?
    a. increase
    b. no change
    c. decrease
    d. cannot be predicted

18. All of the following murmurs will increase in intensity with expiration except:
    a. mitral regurgitation
    b. valvular aortic stenosis
    c. aortic regurgitation
    d. pulmonary regurgitation

19. All of the following murmurs will decrease in intensity with expiration except:
    a. mitral regurgitation
    b. valvular pulmonic stenosis
    c. pulmonary regurgitation
    d. tricuspid regurgitation

ANSWERS - Section 4G

Review practice answers

1. decrease
2. True
3. increase
4. increase
5. False
6. True
7. increase
8. increase
9. decrease
10. decrease
11. decrease
12. True
13. increase
14. decrease
15. decrease
16. True
17. True
18. True
19. increases
20. increases
21. False
22. decreases
23. increase
24. decrease

Board review answers

1.	c	14.	a
2.	c	15.	b
3.	a	16.	a
4.	c	17.	c
5.	c	18.	d
6.	a	19.	a
7.	c		
8.	c		
9.	d		
10.	a		
11.	d		
12.	d		
13.	a		

SECTION 4H
Normal Heart Sound Generation and Timing

There are two normal heart sounds. The first heart sound, S1, is produced by the closure of the atrioventricular valves, primarily the mitral, with a difficult to hear tricuspid component following the closure of the mitral valve. S1 occurs at the onset of the QRS complex. S2 is produced by the closure of the semilunar valves, the aortic valve first and then the pulmonic. Aortic valve closure normally produces the loudest component of S2. S2 occurs at the end of the electrocardiogram T wave.

S1

As the ventricles begin to contract, pressure within the ventricles rapidly exceeds atrial pressure, thus closing the atrioventricular valves. S1 occurs with the onset of the QRS complex. Mitral valve closure occurs before tricuspid valve closure. S1 may be best heard as a single sound at the cardiac apex. The splitting of S1, mitral valve closure followed by tricuspid valve closure, is difficult to hear but may be attempted at the lower left sternal border or subxyphoid area.

S2

As the ventricles eject most of their blood, their pressure begins to fall. When ventricular pressure falls below arterial pressure near the end of ventricular systole, the semilunar valves close. S2 corresponds to semilunar valve closure which occurs at the end of the T wave of the electrocardiogram. Aortic valve closure occurs before pulmonic valve closure. Physiologic splitting of S2, aortic valve closure followed by pulmonic valve closure, may be heard with the stethescope placed in the left upper sternal border area. The interval between aortic valve closure and pulmonic valve closure is affected by respiration with an increase in the interval during inspiration and a decrease in the interval with expiration.

HEART SOUNDS

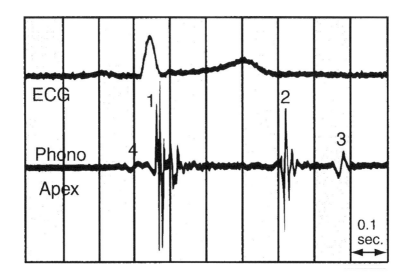

REVIEW PRACTICE - Section 4H

1. The two normal heart sounds are S____ and S____.

2. S1 is caused by the closure of first the _____ valve and then followed by the _____ valve.

3. The major component of the S1 heart sound is closure of the _____ valve.

4. S2 is caused by the closure of first the _____ valve followed by the _____ valve.

5. The major component of the S2 heart sound is the closure of the _____ valve.

6. True or False: S1 occurs when ventricular pressure exceeds atrial pressure with the onset of ventricular systole.

7. True or False: S1 normally occurs at the onset of the QRS complex.

8. True or False: Tricuspid valve closure occurs before mitral valve closure.

9. True or False: S2 occurs when ventricular pressure falls below arterial pressure.

10 True or False: S2 occurs at the end of the P wave of the electrocardiogram.

11. True or False: Aortic valve closure normally occurs after pulmonic valve closure.

12. True or False: Normal physiologic splitting of S2 may best be heard with a stethescope at the upper left sternal border.

13. True or False: S1 and S2 are normally heard throughout the precordium.

14. True or False: S1 is best heard at the cardiac apex.

15. True or False: S2 is best heard at the cardiac base.

BOARD REVIEW QUESTIONS - Section 4H

1. The two normal heart sounds are:
    a. S1, S2
    b. S3, S4
    c. loud S1, opening snap
    d. ejection click, friction rub

2. S1 is caused by:
    a. closure of the atrioventricular valves
    b. opening of the atrioventricular valves
    c. closure of the semilunar valves
    d. opening of the semilunar valves

3. The major component of the S1 heart sound is closure of the:
    a. aortic valve
    b. mitral valve
    c. pulmonic valve
    d. tricuspid valve

4. S2 is caused by the:
    a. closure of the atrioventricular valves
    b. opening of the atrioventricular valves
    c. closure of the semilunar valves
    d. opening of the semilunar valves

5. S1 occurs when:
    a. ventricular pressure exceeds arterial pressure
    b. ventricular pressure exceeds atrial pressure
    c. arterial pressure exceeds ventricular pressure
    d. ventricular pressure exceeds arterial pressure

6. According to the electrocardiogram, S1 coincides with the:
    a. A wave
    b. QRS complex
    c. T wave
    d. u wave

7. Compared to the mitral valve, tricuspid valve closure normally occurs:
    a. before
    b. simultaneous
    c. after
    d. varies

8. S2 occurs when:
   a. ventricular pressure falls below atrial pressure
   b. atrial pressure exceeds ventricular pressure
   c. ventricular pressure falls below arterial pressure
   d. arterial pressure exceeds ventricular pressure

9. In relation to the electrocardiogram, S2 occurs at the end of the:
   a. A wave
   b. QRS complex
   c. T wave
   d. u wave

10. Compared to the aortic valve, the pulmonary valve normally closes:
   a. before
   b. simultaneous
   c. after
   d. varies

ANSWERS - Section 4H

Review practice answers

1. 1, 2
2. mitral, tricuspid
3. mitral
4. aortic, pulmonic
5. aortic
6. True
7. True
8. False
9. True
10. False
11. False
12. True
13. True
14. True
15. True

Board review answers

1. a
2. a
3. b
4. c
5. b
6. b
7. c
8. c
9. c
10. c

SECTION 4I
Cardiovascular Circulation

1. NORMAL METABOLIC NEEDS

The normal metabolic demands of the body are supplied by an interaction of the heart, great vessels, arteries, capillaries and veins. The primary function of the heart is to supply adequate energy for the delivery of oxygenated blood and substrates to metabolizing tissues and for the removal of carbon dioxide and heat.

2. COMPONENT PARTS OF THE CIRCULATION

The component parts of the circulation include the aorta, peripheral arteries, arterioles, capillaries, venules and veins. The walls of an artery consists of three layers. The inner layer is the tunica intima. The middle, thickest layer is the tunica media. The outer layer is the tunica adventitia. The vasa vasorum provides oxygen and nutrients to the vessel walls. The veins have the same three layers but are thinner.

Aorta: The great vessel that conducts blood from the left ventricle to the peripheral arteries.

Peripheral arteries: Peripheral arteries transport oxygenated blood from the aorta to the various tissues of the body.

Arterioles: The arterioles are the last branches of the arterial system and act as control valves by releasing blood to the capillaries. The muscular wall of the arteriole is capable of undergoing large changes in caliber and thus is able to alter blood flow to the capillaries.

Capillaries: The entire arterial system ends with the capillaries which is a vast network of over 10 billion microscopic vessels that function to provide oxygen nutrients, carbon dioxide and waste exchange.

Venules: These veins collect blood from the capillaries.

Veins: The function of the veins is to conduct blood from the peripheral tissues to the heart.

REVIEW PRACTICE - Section 4I

1. True or False: The primary function of the heart is to provide for the metabolic demands of the body.

2. The component parts of the circulation include the aorta, peripheral arteries, arterioles, capillaries, venules and _____.

3. The inner layer of a vessel is called the tunica _____.

4. The middle, thickest layer of a vessel is the tunica _____.

5. The outer layer of a vessel is called the tunica _____.

6. The tiny vessels that supply oxygen and nutrients to the vessel walls is called the _____ _____.

7. The _____ conducts oxygenated blood from the left ventricle to the peripheral arteries.

8. The _____ arteries transport oxygenated blood from the aorta to the various tissues of the body.

9. The _____ are the last branches of the arterial system which act as control valves through which blood is metered into the capillaries.

10. The _____ are the end point of the cardiovascular system and provide for the exchange of oxygen, nutrients, carbon dioxide and waste.

11. The _____ collect deoxygenated blood from the capillaries.

12. The _____ main function is to conduct deoxygenated blood from the peripheral tissues to the heart.

BOARD REVIEW QUESTIONS - Section 4I

1. Which one of the following organs has as its primary function to provide for the metabolic demands of the body?
    a. heart
    b. lungs
    c. brain
    d. kidneys

2. All of the following are component parts of the circulation except:
    a. arterioles
    b. capillaries
    c. venules
    d. vasa vasorum

3. The inner layer of a vessel wall is the tunica:
    a. adventitia
    b. media
    c. intima
    d. vasa vasorum

4. The middle, thickest layer of a vessel wall is the tunica:
    a. intima
    b. media
    c. adventitia
    d. vasa vasorum

5. The outer layer of a vessel wall is called the tunica:
    a. adventitia
    b. media
    c. intima
    d. vasa vasorum

6. Which of the following provides oxygenated blood and nutrients to blood vessel walls?
    a. tunica intima
    b. tunica media
    c. tunica adventitia
    d. vasa vasorum

7. Which of the following arteries conducts blood from the left ventricle to the peripheral arteries?
    a. aorta
    b. arterioles
    c. capillaries
    d. vasa vasorum

8. Which of the following arteries conducts blood from the aorta to the various organs of the body?
    a. aorta
    b. peripheral arteries
    c. arterioles
    d. capillaries

9. Which of the following arteries act as control valves through which blood is metered into the capillaries?
    a. aorta
    b. peripheral arteries
    c. arterioles
    d. capillaries

10. Which of the following provide for the exchange of oxygen, nutrients, carbon dioxide and waste?
    a. aorta
    b. peripheral arteries
    c. arterioles
    d. capillaries

11. Which of the following vessels collect deoxygenated blood from the capillaries?
    a. veins
    b. venules
    c. vasa vasorum
    d. vena cava

12. Which of the following vessels conducts deoxygenated blood from the peripheral tissues to the heart?
    a. veins
    b. venules
    c. vasa vasorum
    d. vena cava

ANSWERS - Section 4I

Review practice answers

1. True
2. veins
3. intima
4. media
5. adventitia
6. vasa vasorum
7. aorta
8. peripheral
9. arterioles
10. capillaries
11. venules
12. veins

Board review answers

1. a
2. d
3. c
4. b
5. a
6. d
7. a
8. b
9. c
10. d
11. b
12. a

3. CONTROL MECHANISMS

Cardiac performance can be reflected by any number of measurements (i.e. stroke volume, cardiac output) and is influenced by preload, afterload, myocardial contractility and heart rate as well as the autonomic nervous system.

Preload: The amount of diastolic filling of the heart. Preload may be measured clinically by end-diastolic pressure or volume via the pulmonary wedge pressure or central venous pressure. To a certain physiologic limit, an increase in end-diastolic pressure or volume (preload) will enhance cardiac contractility. This is known as the length-tension relationship or the Frank-Starling law of the heart. An increase in preload is associated with chamber dilatation.

Afterload: The resistance the ventricle faces while ejecting blood. Afterload is dependent upon the resistance of the semilunar valves, blood viscosity and arterial blood pressure. An increase in afterload, such as seen in semilunar valve stenosis, polycythemia or systemic/pulmonary hypertension will increase the work of the heart and will cause the ventricle to contract more slowly. This is known as the force-velocity relationship. In patients with poor cardiac function, an increase in afterload will decrease cardiac performance. Right ventricular afterload is assessed clinically by obtaining the mean pulmonary artery pressure. Left ventricular afterload is assessed clinically by obtaining the mean arterial pressure. An increase in afterload is associated with chamber hypertrophy.

Contractility: Myocardial contractility is the inherent property of the heart muscle's ability to contract. Myocardial ischemia or infarction impairs the inherent property of the myocardium to contract, and therefore cardiac performance is decreased. Myocardial contractility may also be altered by the sympathetic and parasympathetic nervous systems, blood gases, pH, hormones, preload and afterload.

Heart rate: Cardiac performance may be enhanced by a decrease in heart rate because it allows for greater diastolic filling.

The autonomic nervous system may influence heart rate because the sympathetic and parasympathetic nervous system innervate the sinoatrial node and the atrioventricular node. The sympathetic nervous system may increase excitability (bathomotropic effect), pacemaker firing rate (chronotropic effect), conduction speed (dromotropic effect) and contractility (inotropic effect). The parasympathetic nervous system, which originates from the X cranial (vagus) nerve, decreases excitability, pacemaker firing rate, conduction speed and contractility. Normally the parasympathetic nervous system predominates. This may be observed in cardiac transplant patients whose parasympathetic system (vagus nerve) has been disrupted. Cardiac transplant patients have increased heart rate.

REVIEW PRACTICE - Section 4I

1. Cardiac performance may be influenced by 1._____, 2._____, 3._____ and/or 4._____ _____.

2. The amount of ventricular diastolic filling is referred to as: _____.

3. True or False: Preload may be evaluated by measuring end-diastolic pressure or end-diastolic volume.

4. True or False: An increase in preload may enhance cardiac performance according to the Frank-Starling law of the heart.

5. The resistance a ventricle faces as it ejects blood is called: _____.

6. True or False: Pulmonary hypertension may cause a decrease in cardiac performance due to the increase in afterload.

7. The inherent property of the heart to contract is referred to as myocardial: _____.

8. True or False: A myocardial infarction may decrease cardiac performance because of its effect on myocardial contractility.

9. True or False: Heart rate may enhance or decrease cardiac performance.

10. The _____ nervous system enhances excitability, pacemaker firing rate, conduction speed and contractility.

11. The _____ nervous system decreases excitability, pacemaker firing rate, conduction speed and contractility.

12. True or False: The sympathetic nervous system will increase heart rate and the force of contraction.

13. True or False: The parasympathetic nervous system will decrease heart rate and the force of contractility.

14. True or False: Normally the parasympathetic nervous system predominates over the sympathetic nervous system.

15. The term _____ refers to excitability.

16. The term_____ refers to the pacemaker firing rate.

17. The term _____ refers to cardiac cell conduction speed.

18. The term _____ refers to contractility.

19. True or False: Any cardiac performance measurement (i.e. stroke volume, cardiac output) is influenced by the interrelationship of preload, afterload, the state of myocardial contractility heart rate and the autonomic nervous system.

BOARD REVIEW QUESTIONS - Section 4I

1. All of the following may affect cardiac performance except:
    a. preload
    b. afterload
    c. contractility
    d. blood velocity

2. The amount of ventricular diastolic filling is called:
    a. preload
    b. afterload
    c. contractility
    d. heart rate

3. The amount of preload may be measured clinically by:
    a. atrial diastole
    b. ventricular end-diastolic pressure
    c. arterial end-systolic volume
    d. measuring myocardial cell length

4. According to the Frank-Starling law, an increase in preload may have which effect on cardiac performance?
    a. increase
    b. no change
    c. decreased
    d. cannot be determined

5. The resistance a ventricle encounters during ventricular systole is called:
    a. preload
    b. afterload
    c. contractility
    d. heart rate

6. What effect will an increase in afterload have on cardiac performance?
    a. increase
    b. no change
    c. decrease
    d. cannot be determined

7. All of the following will increase afterload except:
    a. semilunar valve stenosis
    b. anemia
    c. pulmonary hypertension
    d. systemic hypertension

8. The inherent property of the ventricle to contract is called:
    a. preload
    b. afterload
    c. contractility
    d. heart rate

9. Which of the following will directly affect myocardial contractility?
    a. mitral stenosis
    b. myocardial infarction
    c. cor triatriatum
    d. tricuspid stenosis

10. According to the Frank-Starling law of the heart, a decrease in heart rate may have which effect on cardiac performance?
    a. increase
    b. no change
    c. decrease
    d. cannot be predicted

11. Which of the following will enhance cardiac cell excitability, pacemaker firing rate, conduction speed and contractility?
    a. parasympathetic nervous system
    b. sympathetic nervous system
    c. autonomic nervous system
    d. preload

12. Which of the following will decrease cardiac cell excitability, pacemaker firing rate, conduction speed and contractility?
    a. parasymapthetic nervous system
    b. sympathetic nervous system
    c. autonomic nervous system
    d. afterload

13. The term bathomotropic refers to:
    a. excitability
    b. pacemaker firing rate
    c. rate of conduction
    d. contractility

14. The term chronotropic refers to:
    a. excitability
    b. pacemaker firing rate
    c. rate of conduction
    d. contractility

CHAPTER 4 (UNIT FOUR) - CARDIAC PHYSIOLOGY

15. The term dromotropic refers to:
    a. excitability
    b. pacemaker firing rate
    c. rate of conduction
    d. contractility

16. The term inotropic refers to:
    a. excitability
    b. pacemaker firing rate
    c. rate of conduction
    d. contractility

ANSWERS - Section 4I

Review practice answers

1. preload, afterload, contractility, heart rate
2. preload
3. True
4. True
5. afterload
6. True
7. contractility
8. True
9. True
10. sympathetic
11. parasympathetic
12. True
13. True
14. True
15. bathomotropic
16. chronotropic
17. dromotropic
18. inotropic
19. True

Board review answers

1. d
2. a
3. b
4. a
5. b
6. c
7. b
8. c
9. b
10. a
11. b
12. a
13. a
14. b
15. c
16. d

4. CORONARY CIRCULATION

Coronary artery blood flow occurs predominantly during ventricular diastole. The amount of coronary blood flow is affected by the following factors:

Coronary artery disease: A stenosis of at least 70% is considered significant because it will lead to a decrease in blood flow distally. Additionally, a significant coronary artery stenosis may cause the artery distal to the lesion to dilate causing the coronary artery to lose its reserve capacity for further dilation in the face of increased oxygen demand.

Aortic diastolic blood pressure: Because the aortic valve cusps partially occlude the coronary ostia during ventricular systole, coronary artery blood flow is predominantly diastolic. A decrease in aortic diastolic blood pressure, such as may occur in severe aortic regurgitation, may decrease the amount of coronary blood flow.

Left ventricular diastolic pressure: An increase in left ventricular diastolic pressure may decrease the amount of coronary artery blood flow.

Heart rate: An increase in heart rate will shorten ventricular diastole and therefore may decrease the amount of coronary artery blood flow.

Collateral vessels: Collateral coronary artery blood flow may be established in patients with ischemic occlusion, thus preserving the amount of coronary blood flow.

Metabolic factors: Neurohormonal responses, autoregulatory receptor activity and certain drugs will affect coronary circulation.

REVIEW PRACTICE - Section 4I

163

1. Coronary artery blood flow predominantly occurs during ventricular _____.

2. Significant coronary artery stenosis is considered to be present when the the vessel diameter is decreased by at least _____%.

3. True or False: A change in aortic diastolic blood pressure may affect coronary artery circulation.

4. True or False: A change in left ventricular diastolic pressure may affect coronary artery circulation.

5. True or False: A change in heart rate may affect coronary artery circulation.

6. True or False: Collateral coronary circulation may be established in patients with ischemic occlusion thus improving coronary circulation.

7. True or False: Certain physiologic and pharmacological factors influence the degree of coronary circulation.

BOARD REVIEW QUESTIONS - Section 4I

1. Coronary artery blood flow occurs predominantly during:
   a. atrial systole
   b. ventricular diastole
   c. ventricular systole
   d. isovolumic contraction

2. Significant coronary artery disease is present when the percent decrease in coronary artery diameter is at least:
   a. 30%
   b. 50%
   c. 70%
   d. 90%

3. Which of the following pathologies would most likely affect coronary artery circulation?
   a. mitral stenosis
   b. tricuspid stenosis
   c. aortic regurgitation
   d. tricuspid regurgitation

4. An increase in left ventricular diastolic pressure may have which effect on coronary circulation?
   a. increase
   b. no change
   c. decrease
   d. cannot be predicted

5. An increase in heart rate will have which effect on coronary circulation?
   a. increase
   b. no change
   c. decrease
   d. cannot be predicted

6. The establishment of collateral circulation will have which effect on coronary circulation?
   a. increase
   b. no change
   c. decrease
   d. cannot be predicted

ANSWERS - Section 4I

Review practice answers

1. diastole
2. 70
3. True
4. True
5. True
6. True
7. True

Board review answers

1. b
2. c
3. c
4. c
5. c
6. a

5. PROPERTIES OF BLOOD: COMPOSITION

Blood has two distinct fractions: formed elements (blood cells) and plasma. Formed elements constitute 38% to 52% while plasma constitutes approximately 55%.

The following are the formed elements of blood:

Red blood cells (erythrocytes): Red blood cells are bioconcave discs that are produced in the red bone marrow via a process called erythropoesis. The red blood cell carries the pigment called hemoglobin which combines with and transports oxygen. Red blood cells constitute approximately 45% of the formed elements of blood.

White blood cells (leukocytes): White blood cells are a part of the body's immune system. White blood cells constitute approximately 1% of the formed elements.

Platelets (thrombocyctes): Platelets play an important role in blood coagulation. Platelets make up approximately 1% of the formed elements.

Plasma: Plasma is the fluid in which the formed elements are suspended. Plasma carries proteins, electrolytes, enzymes, hormones, cholesterol and uric acid. Plasma constitutes approximately 55% of blood.

Important terms

Hematocrit: refers to the percentage of red blood cells present.

Plasmacrit: refers to the percentage of plasma present.

Polycythemia: is the abnormal increase in the number of red blood cells

Anemia: is the abnormal decrease in the number of red blood cells

Leukocytosis: is an abnormal increase in the number of white blood cells

Leukopenia: is an abnormal decrease in the number of white blood cells

REVIEW PRACTICE - Section 4I

1.   Blood has two distinct fractions: _____ elements and _____.

2.   The three components that make up the formed elements of blood are: 1._____blood cells, 2._____blood cells and 3._____.

3.   Red blood cells are also referred to as:_____.

4.   White blood cells are also referred to as: _____.

5.   Platelets are also referred to as: _____.

6.   _____ is the fluid in which the formed elements are suspended.

7.   True or False: Plasma carries proteins, enzymes, hormones, cholesterol and uric acid.

8.   _____ is the term used to describe the percentage of red blood cells present.

9.   _____ is term that expresses the percentage of plasma present.

10.   _____ is an increase in red blood cells.

11.   _____ is a decrease in the number of red blood cells.

12.   _____ is an increase in the number of white blood cells.

13.   _____ is a decrease in the number of white blood cells.

14.   _____ is the production of red blood cells.

BOARD REVIEW QUESTIONS - Section 4I

1. The two distinct fractions of blood are plasma and:
    a. red blood cells
    b. white blood cells
    c. platelets
    d. formed elements

2. All of the following are a component of the formed elements of blood except:
    a. red blood cells
    b. white blood cells
    c. platelets
    d. plasma

3. Red blood cells are also referred to as:
    a. plasma
    b. erythrocytes
    b. leukocytes
    d. thrombocytes

4. White blood cells are also referred to as:
    a. plasma
    b. erythrocytes
    c. leukocytes
    d. thrombocytes

5. Platelets are also referred to as:
    a. plasma
    b. erythrocytes
    c. leukocytes
    d. thrombocytes

6. The fluid that carries the formed elements of blood is called:
    a. platelets
    b. erythrocytes
    c. leukocytes
    d. plasma

7. The percentage of red blood cells present is called:
    a. anemia
    b. plasmacrit
    c. hematocrit
    d. polycthemia

8. The percentage of plasma present is:
    a. hematocrit
    b. polycythemia
    c. plasmacrit
    d. leukopenia

9. An increase in the number of red blood cells is:
    a. anemia
    b. polycythemia
    c. leukopenia
    d. hematocrit

10. A decrease in the number of red blood cells is:
    a. anemia
    b. polycythemia
    c. leukopenia
    d. plasmacrit

11. An increase in the number of white blood cells is:
    a. anemia
    b. plasmacrit
    c. leukopenia
    d. leukocytosis

12. A decrease in the number of white blood cells is:
    a. anemia
    b. hematocrit
    c. leukopenia
    d. leukocytosis

ANSWERS - Section 4I

Review practice answers

1. formed, plasma
2. red, white, platelets
3. erythrocytes
4. leukocytes
5. thrombocytes
6. plasma
7. True
8. hematocrit
9. plasmacrit
10. polycythemia
11. anemia
12. leukocytosis
13. leukopenia
14. erythropoeisis

Board review answers

1. d
2. d
3. b
4. c
5. d
6. d
7. c
8. c
9. b
10. a
11. d
12. c

CHAPTER FIVE
CARDIAC EVALUATION METHODS

SECTION A.   Symptoms of Cardiac Diseases and
                               Common Causes

SECTION B.   Physical Examination and Signs

SECTION C.   Electrocardiography (EKG)

SECTION D.   Phonocardiography

SECTION E.   Cardiac Catheterization

SECTION F.   Other Diagnostic Modalities

SECTION 5A
Symptoms of Cardiac Diseases and Common Causes

Pulsus alternans: Pulsus alternans refers to a pattern in which there is regular alteration of the pressure pulse amplitude, despite a regular rhythm. It is associated with very poor left ventricular systolic function.

Pulsus bisferiens: A bisferiens pulse is characterized by two systolic peaks. It is associated with severe aortic regurgitation or hypertrophic obstructive cardiomyopathy.

Pulsus paradoxus: Pulsus paradoxus is an exaggeration of the normal decrease in systolic blood pressure. To be considered abnormal, the drop must be greater than 10 mm Hg. It is associated with cardiac tamponade.

Pulsus parvus et tardus: Pulsus parvus et tardus denotes a small, weak, late peaking pulse. It is associated with valvular aortic stenosis.

Displacement of the point of maximal impulse: Normally the point of maximal impulse measures less than 2 to 3 cm in diameter and is confined to a single intercostal space. Displacement downward and to the left usually indicates an enlarged heart.

Edema: Edema may be rated on a scale from 1+ to 4+. 1+ pitting edema is a barely detectable pit while 4+ edema is a deep and persistent pit approximately 1 inch deep. Brawny edema is considered present when pitting is impossible to demonstrate because the subcutaneous tissue has developed fibrosis. Peripheral edema is associated with right heart failure. Pulmonary edema is associated with left heart failure.

Left parasternal lift: A left parasternal lift is due to anterior displacement of the right ventricle due to a large left atrium. It may be found in patients with severe, chronic mitral regurgitation.

Left ventricular thrust: Left ventricular hypertrophy results in an exaggerated amplitude and duration of the normal left ventricular thrust. It is associated with aortic stenosis, hypertrophic cardiomyopathy, systemic hypertension.

Left ventricular systolic bulge: A left ventricular systolic bulge is a larger than normal area of pulsation of the left ventricular apex. It is associated with left ventricular aneurysm.

Thrills: Thrills are palpable manifestations of loud, harsh murmurs with low frequency components. Thrills are associated with aortic and pulmonic stenosis as well as ventricular septal defect.

Angina: Angina pectoris is chest pain due to myocardial ischemia. Chest pain in general may indicate the presence of pericarditis, dissecting aortic aneurysm, pulmonary embolus, pneumothorax, gastrointestinal problems or acute anxiety.

Cachexia: Cachexia is a state of ill health, malnutrition and wasting and is associated with long standing heart disease.

Clubbing: Clubbing is a condition that affects the fingers and toes. It is a lateral and longitudinal curvature of the nails accompanied by soft tissue enlargement. Clubbing is associated with cyanotic heart disease.

Congestive heart failure: Congestive heart failure is a syndrome or clinical condition resulting from failure of the heart to maintain adequate circulation of blood. The causes of congestive heart failure include myocardial dysfunction, pressure overload, volume overload, diastolic dysfunction or increased metabolic demands.

Cor pulmonale: Cor pulmonale is defined as a combination of hypertrophy and dilatation of the right ventricle caused by pulmonary hypertension that results from a process intrinsic to the lung.

Cyanosis: Cyanosis is the bluish discoloration of the skin and mucous membranes. Cyanosis is associated with right to left cardiac shunts or pulmonary disease.

Dyspnea: Dyspnea is an abnormal uncomfortable awareness of breathing. It is the main symptom for cardiac and pulmonary disease. There are two types of dyspnea that may indicate a cardiac origin. Orthopnea is dyspnea while lying flat and is associated with congestive heart failure. Paroxysmal nocturnal dyspnea is dyspnea that interrupts sleep. It usually is caused by pulmonary edema secondary to left ventricular failure.

Edema: Edema is the accumulation of fluid in cells, tissues or cavities. Hypertension, left ventricular failure, and increased venous pressure secondary to right heart failure are possible causes of cardiac related edema.

Fever/chills: A history of fever and chills is common in patients with a history of infective endocarditis.

Hepatomegaly: Hepatomegaly is enlargement of the liver and is associated with right heart failure.

Hemoptysis: Hemoptysis is the appearance of blood in the sputum due to pulmonary hemmorhage. Hemoptysis is associated with mitral stenosis.

Jugular venous distention: Jugular venous distention is a term widely used to indicate high pressures in the right heart.

Nocturia: Nocturia is excessive urination at night and is associated with congestive heart failure.

Palpitations: Palpitations are the uncomfortable awareness of the heart beating. Palpitations may be caused by cardiac arrhythmias, smoking, exercise, stress or excessive consumption of beverages containing caffeine.

Pectus excavatum/carinatum: Pectus carinatum is a forward projection of the sternum. Pectus excavatum is the backward displacement of the lower sternum and xiphoid cartilage causing a hollow area over the lower sternum. Thoracic cage abnormalities are associated with Marfan's syndrome and mitral valve prolapse.

Syncope: Syncope, faintness and light headedness are frequent problems in patients with cardiac disease. Syncope refers to a transient loss of consciousness. Cardiac causes of syncope include arrhythmia, angina, myocardial infarction, left ventricular outflow tract obstruction, hypotension and pacemaker failure.

SECTION 5B

Physical Examination and Signs
1. GENERAL PHYSICAL APPEARANCE AND PATIENT HISTORY

The cardiac physical examination includes inspection, palpation, percussion and auscultation.

Inspection

Inspection includes an assessment of the patient's distress level, level of consciousness, skin and mucous membranes, jugular veins, carotid artery pulsations, anterior chest and extremities.

Palpation

Palpation is utilized to assess a patient's arterial pulses, extremities and anterior chest. Cardiac palpation is performed to evaluate the:

> apical impulse
> right ventricle
> pulmonary artery
> left ventricular motions
> presence/absence of thrills

Percussion

Percussion refers to the technique of tapping on a surface to determine the underlying structure. The examiner places the middle finger of the left hand firmly against the chest wall and uses the tip of the right middle finger to strike a quick, sharp blow to the terminal phalanx of the left finger on the chest wall. Percussion of the heart is utilized to determine heart size, dextrocardia or tension pneumothorax.

Auscultation

Cardiac auscultation is the process of utilizing a stethescope to detect heart sounds and murmurs. Cardiac auscultation should be carried out in an organized manner by listening in the aortic area first followed by the pulmonic area, tricuspid area and the mitral area. The seven rules for cardiac auscultation are:
1. Concentrate on the first heart sound (S1)
2. Concentrate on the second heart sound (S2)
3. Listen for extra sounds during ventricular systole
4. Listen for extra sounds during ventricular diastole
5. Listen for systolic murmurs
6. Listen for diastolic murmurs
7. Listen for murmurs or heart sounds which have systolic and diastolic components such as pericardial friction rubs.

REVIEW PRACTICE - Section 5A and 5B

1. _____ _____ is chest pain due to myocardial ischemia.

2. Check the following if associated with chest pain:

   _____ pericarditis

   _____ dissecting aortic aneurysm

   _____ pulmonary embolus

   _____ pneumothorax

   _____ esophageal spasm

   _____ hiatal hernia

   _____ peptic ulcer

   _____ acute anxiety

3. _____ is a state of ill health that may be caused by long standing heart disease.

4. _____ is the lateral and longitudinal curvature of the nailbeds and is associated with congenital heart disease.

5. _____ heart failure is the inability of the heart to meet the metabolic demands of the body.

6. Congestive heart failure may be caused by myocardial _____, _____ overload, _____ overload or _____ dysfunction.

7. _____ _____ is right heart failure due to intrinsic pulmonary disease.

8. _____ is the bluish discoloration of the skin associated with a right to left cardiac shunt.

9. _____ is shortness of breath associated with cardiac or pulmonary disease.

10. _____ is dyspnea while lying flat and is associated with congestive heart failure.

11. _____ _____ dyspnea is dyspnea that interrupts sleep and is associated with pulmonary edema secondary to left ventricular failure.

12. _____ is the accumulation of fluid in the cells, tissues or cavities due to ventricular failure.

13. _____ and _____ are associated with infective endocarditis.

14. _____ is the enlargement of the liver associated with right heart failure.

15. _____ is the coughing or spitting up of blood associated with mitral stenosis.

16. _____ _____ distention indicates high right heart pressures.

17. _____ is excessive urination at night associated with mitral stenosis or left heart failure.

18. _____ are the uncomfortable awareness of the heart beating and are associated with arrhythmias, smoking, exercise, stress or excessive consumption of beverages containing caffeine.

19. _____ _____ is the forward projection of the sternum.

20. _____ _____ is the backward displacement of the lower sternum.

21. True or False: Thoracic cage abnormalities such as kyphosis, pectus carinatum and pectus excavatum are rarely found in patients with Marfan's syndrome or patients with mitral valve prolapse.

22. _____ is the temporary loss of consciousness associated with arrhythmia, angina, myocardial infarction, left ventricular outflow tract obstruction, hypotension and pacemaker failure.

23. _____ _____ is the increase and decrease of the pulse associated with poor left systolic ventricular function.

24. _____ _____ is two pulses during one systole associated with hypertrophic cardiomyopathy.

25. _____ _____ et _____ is a small, late rising pulse associated with aortic stenosis.

26. True or False: Downward displacement of the heart usually indicates an enlarged heart.

27. True or False: Pitting edema may be rated as mild (1+) to severe (4+).

28. The left parasternal _____ is caused by the anterior displacement of the right ventricle due to an enlarged left atrium.

29. True or False: A left ventricular thrust is associated with left ventricular hypertrophy.

30. True or False: A left ventricular systolic bulge is associated with left ventricular aneurysm.

31. A _____ is a palpable murmur.

32. The physical examination of the heart includes, _____, _____, _____ and _____.

33. True or False: Percussion may be used to determine cardiac size, dextrocardia or tension pneumothorax.

34. Check the following if considered a rule for cardiac auscultation:
    _____ concentrate on S1
    _____ concentrate on S2
    _____ listen for extra heart sounds during ventricular systole
    _____ listen for extra heart sounds during ventricular diastole
    _____ listen for systolic murmurs
    _____ listen for diastolic murmurs
    _____ listen for heart sounds or murmurs which have a systolic and diastolic component

CHAPTER 5 (UNIT FIVE) - CARDIAC EVALUATION METHODS

BOARD REVIEW QUESTIONS - Section 5A and 5B

CASE ONE

History

A 48 year old male presents to the emergency room with a complaint of several hours of chest discomfort. He has no previous history of heart disease. His risk factors include a 25 year history of smoking and a father with coronary artery disease.

Physical Examination

Blood pressure is 100/60, pulse is 77 bpm. He is pale and diaphoretic. The jugular veins are distended. The lungs are clear by CXR. There is an S4 at the xyphoid area without murmurs. The EKG demonstrates ST segment elevation in leads II, III, and AVF.

The diagnosis is:
      a.   mitral valve prolapse
      b.   infective endocarditis
      c.   coronary artery disease
      d.   acute mitral regurgitation

CASE TWO

History

A 69 year old female presents with several hours of substernal chest pain.

Physical Examination

Blood pressure is 133/75, pulse is 99 bpm. There is an S4. The patient is treated for acute myocardial infarction. On the third day of her hospital stay, she reports respiratory difficulty to the nurse. Blood pressure is 88/40, pulse is 158 bpm. There is no pulsus paradoxus nor jugular venous distention. There is a systolic thrill palpable at the lower left sternal border with a V/VI systolic murmur radiating along the left sternal border. The EKG demonstrates no new findings.

The diagnosis:
      a.   pericardial effusion
      b.   cardiac tamponade
      c.   ventricular septal defect
      d.   myocardial infarction

CASE THREE

History

A 10 year old Chinese girl presents with fever and joint swelling of 8 days duration.

Physical Examination

A thin, underdeveloped female presents with a blood pressure of 122/68, heart rate is 86 bpm. There is a grade 3/6 harsh holosystolic murmur heard best at the apex. There also is a 2/6 early diastolic decresendo murmur detected at the left sternal border. An S3 is present. The EKG demonstrates 1st degree AV block. The CXR is normal.

The diagnosis is:
   a.   acute tricuspid regurgitation
   b.   cardiac tamponade
   c.   acute rheumatic fever
   d.   atrial septal defect

CASE FOUR

History

A 44 year old male presents with a fever of 12 days duration and increasing shortness of breath. There is no history of heart disease in the family. He had a routine teeth cleaning performed 5 weeks prior to presenting.

Physical Examination

Blood pressure is 146/55, pulse is 122 bpm. The left ventricular impulse is hyperdynamic and palpable at the 6th intercostal space 1.5 cm to the left of the midclavicular line. There is a 4/6 early diastolic decrescendo murmur heard at the left upper and mid sternal border. There is a 2/6 systolic ejection murmur heard at the right upper sternal border. The CXR demonstrates cardiomegaly. The EKG is normal.

The diagnosis is:
   a.   acute rheumatic fever
   b.   aortic valve endocarditis
   c.   ruptured papillary muscle
   d.   aortic dissection

CASE FIVE

History

A 68 year old male with a history of a heart murmur presents with a complaint of fatigue and dyspnea. Five years ago he was told he had a click and a heart valve that leaked a bit.

Physical Examination

Blood pressure is 133/80 and heart rate pulse is 92 bpm. There is no jugular venous distention. The left ventricular impulse is between the 5th and 6th intercostal space. There is a left parasternal lift and a systolic thrill at the apex. Grade 3/6 holosystolic murmur is heard at the apex radiating to the axilla. The EKG demonstrates left atrial enlargement. The CXR reveals mild pectus excavatum and cardiomegaly.

The diagnosis is:
- a. infective endocarditis
- b. constrictive pericarditis
- c. cardiac tamponade
- d. mitral valve prolapse

CASE SIX

History

A 21 year old male presents with complaints of fatigue and dyspnea upon exertion. There is no history of rheumatic fever, chest pain, orthopnea or edema. He does complain of palpitations and remembers a doctor told him that his heart sounds were not normal.

Physical Examination

Blood pressure is 150/50 and pulse is 78 bpm. The pulses are noted to be prominent. A hyperdynamic left ventricular impulse is left of the midclavicular line. S1 and S2 are normal. A grade II/VI systolic ejection murmur is heard at the right upper sternal border. A grade IV/VI diastolic decrescendo murmur is heard along the left sternal border. A brisk pulse is noted in the fingers that fades away suddenly. The EKG demonstrates LVH and the CXR shows mild-moderate cardiomegaly.

The diagnosis is:
- a. congenital mitral stenosis
- b. ventricular septal defect
- c. congenital aortic stenosis/regurgitation
- d. tetralogy of Fallot

CASE SEVEN

History

A 78 year old retired steel worker presents with exertional fatigue and dyspnea. He states that while working on his house he experienced chest palpitations. A murmur was detected 15 years ago and 2 years ago a CXR demonstrated mild cardiomegaly.

Physical Examination

Blood pressure is 120/80 with a pulse of 122 and irregular. There is jugular venous distention and the left ventricular impulse is felt 1.5 cm left and the midclavicular line in the 6th intercostal space. There is a grade 3/6 harsh, holosytolic murmur best heard at the apex and radiates to the axilla. The murmur decreases with Valsalva. There is an S3 and no diastolic murmur. Mild pedal edema is present. The EKG demonstrates LVH and atrial fibrillation. The CXR demonstrates moderate cardiomegaly with cephalization of blood flow in the lungs.

The diagnosis is:
- a. dilated cardiomyopathy
- b. hypertrophic cardiomyopathy
- c. restrictive cardiomyopathy
- d. hypertensive cardiomyopathy

CASE EIGHT

History

A 62 year old male presents with an episode of syncope. For the past few months, he has complained about exertional chest pain. He was told that he had a murmur "years ago".

Physical Examination

Blood pressure is 112/83 and the heart rate is 66 bpm. His carotid upstroke is delayed and the amplitude of the carotid pulse is dampened. There is a prominent LV impulse at the 5th intercostal space at the midclavicular line. S1 is normal, S2 is soft. A 4/6 late-peaking systolic ejection murmur is detected best at the right upper sternal border. There is a 2/6 holosystolic murmur heard at the apex and radiates to the axilla. There is a 2/6 early diastolic murmur heard best at the left sternal border. The EKG demonstrates LVH. The CXR is normal.

The diagnosis is:
- a. hypertrophic cardiomyopathy
- b. rheumatic mitral stenosis
- c. severe aortic regurgitation
- d. valvular aortic stenosis

CHAPTER 5 (UNIT FIVE) - CARDIAC EVALUATION METHODS

CASE NINE

History

A 57 year old Hispanic female presents with fatigue, exertional dyspnea and hemoptysis. She has never seen a physician prior to this.

Physical Examination

Blood pressure is 103/68, the pulse is irregular at 133 bpm. S1 is loud, S2 is normal. There is a weak LV impulse and an RV lift along the left sternal border. An opening snap is heard after S2 and a presystolic murmur is detected just prior to vertricular systole. The EKG demonstrates atrial fibrillation. The CXR demonstrates cephalization of flow in the lungs.

The diagnosis is:
- a. rheumatic mitral stenosis
- b. valvular aortic stenosis
- c. aortic aneurysm
- d. infective endocarditis

CASE TEN

History

A 26 year old female musician presents with sharp chest pain that is located closer to the cardiac apex. She states that her heart seems to "skip beats" and she is aware of this during times of stress.

Physical Examination

Blood pressure is 130/80 and the heart rate is 88 bpm. There is a midsystolic, high pitched click at the cardiac apex. A II/VI apical end-systolic murmur is present. The EKG and CXR are normal. A 24-hour ambulatory EKG demonstrated multiple PVC's.

The diagnosis is:
- a. aortic dissection
- b. cardiac tamponade
- c. patent ductus arteriosus
- d. mitral valve prolapse

ANSWERS - Section 5A and 5B

Review practice answers

1. angina pectoris
2. all
3. cachexia
4. clubbing
5. congestive
6. dysfunction, pressure, volume, diastolic
7. cor pulmonale
8. cyanosis
9. dyspnea
10. orthopnea
11. paroxysmal nocturnal
12. edema
13. fever, chills
14. hepatomegaly
15. hemoptysis
16. jugular venous
17. nocturia
18. palpitations
19. pectus carinatum
20. pectus excavatum
21. False
22. syncope
23. pulsus alternans
24. pulsus bisfieriens
25. pulsus parvus et tardus
26. True
27. True
28. lift
29. True
30. True
31. thrill
32. inspection, palpation, percussion, auscultation
33. True
34. all

Board review answers

1. c
2. c
3. c
4. b

5. d
6. c
7. a
8. d
9. a
10. d

CHAPTER 5 (UNIT FIVE) - CARDIAC EVALUATION METHODS

2. CORRELATION OF AUSCULTATORY FINDINGS

The physical examination includes cardiac auscultation. A stethescope with tubing that is 10" to 12" in length should be used. The bell of the stethescope enables the evaluation of low pitched heart sounds. The diaphragm of the stethescope is utilized to evaluate high pitched heart sounds. Aortic valve heart sounds and murmurs are best heard at the right upper sternal border. Pulmonic valve heart sounds and murmurs are best heard at the left upper sternal border. The mitral valve heart sounds and murmurs may be best auscultated at the cardiac apex. The lower left sternal border or subxyphoid area is the best area(s) to listen to tricuspid valve heart sounds and murmurs.

Normal Heart Sounds

S1: The first heart sound (S1) is caused by the closure of the atrioventricular valves at the onset of ventricular systole. The mitral valve closes first and is easily detected followed by tricuspid valve closure which is difficult to hear normally. S1 is heard throughout the precordium but may best be auscultated at the cardiac apex (mitral area) to the lower left sternal border (tricuspid area) with the diaphragm of the stethescope. The mitral valve closure sound is usually greater in intensity than the tricuspid valve closure. S1 is the lub in the lub-dup description of the normal heart sounds and is normally lower pitched than S2.

S2: S2 represents the closure of the semilunar valves at the end of ventricular systole. Aortic valve closure (A2) is usually best heard at the right upper sternal border (aortic area) while the pulmonic valve closure (P2) is best heard at the left upper sternal border (pulmonic area) with the diaphragm of the stethescope. S2 varies with respiration with inspiration splitting S2 and expiration narrowing S2. S2 is the louder of the two heart sounds.

Abnormal Heart Sounds

S3: The S3 is a low pitched heart sound best heard aat the cardiac apex with the bell of the stethescope. S3 is a filling sound as blood accelerates into the ventricles during the rapid filling phase in early diastole with resultant release of energy vibrations from the ventricular walls. A physiologic S3 may be present in persons under the age of 30. If heard in individuals beyond 35 years it is considered pathologic. An S3 may also be called a protodiastolic or ventricular gallop. The following conditions may cause an S3:

    High cardiac output states
    Large left to right shunts
    Anemia
    Valvular regurgitation
    Reduced diastolic filling superimposed on abnormal residual volume or compliance
        (e.g. cardiomyopathy)

S4: The S4 is a low pitched heart sound that occurs in response to atrial systole that is best heard at the cardiac apex with the bell of the stethescope. The S4 is caused by ventricular wall vibrations during the inflow of blood after atrial contraction in patients with abnormal ventricular compliance. The S4 may also be called an atrial or presystolic gallop. The following conditions are associated with an S4:

    Hypertension
    Significant semilunar valve stenosis
    Cardiomyopathy
    Coronary artery disease
    Acute mitral regurgitation

Loud S1: An increase in the intensity of S1 is associated with rheumatic mitral stenosis and is best heard at the cardiac apex with the bell of the stethescope.

Opening snap: The opening snap is most often associated with rheumatic atrioventricular valve stenosis. The opening snap occurs at the maximum initial opening excursion of the atrioventricular valve leaflets, as their limited motion is abruptly checked in early diastole. The mitral valve opening snap is best heard at the cardiac apex with the diaphragm of the stethescope.

Ejection sound or click: Ejection sounds or clicks are high frequency sounds that follow S1 and occur at the time of ventricular ejection. The ejection sound is best heard across the precordium with the diaphragm of the stethescope. The ejection sound commonly indicates the presence of congenital semilunar valve stenosis.

Midsystolic click: The midsystolic click is a high frequency sound that usually occurs during mid to late ventricular systole. The click is best heard at the cardiac apex with the diaphragm of the stethescope. The midsystolic click suggests the presence of mitral valve prolapse.

Fixed split S2: The S2 heart sound is composed of aortic and pulmonic valve closure. Normally the interval between closure varies with respiration. With fixed splitting of S2, the interval is wider with minimal respiratory variation. Fixed split S2 may be best heard at the upper left sternal border with the diaphragm of the stethescope. Fixed split S2 commonly indicates the presence of atrial septal defect.

Pericardial friction rub: The pericardial friction rub is associated with pericarditis and is due to the inflamed visceral and parietal surfaces of the pericardium moving against each other. It may have three components: atrial systole, early ventricular diastole and ventricular systole.

Pericardial knock: A pericardial knock is an early diastolic heart sound associated with constrictive pericarditis. The pericardial knock occurs before the S3 heart sound.

CHAPTER 5 (UNIT FIVE) - CARDIAC EVALUATION METHODS

REVIEW PRACTICE - Section 5B

1. The heart sound S_____ is caused by the closure of the atrioventricular valves.

2. The mitral valve may be best heard at the cardiac _____.

3. True or False: The tricuspid valve may be best heard along the lower left sternal border.

4. The heart sound S_____ is caused by the closure of the semilunar valves.

5. The aortic component of S2 may be best heard at the _____ upper sternal border.

6. The pulmonic component of S2 may be best heard at the _____ upper sternal border.

7. True or False: S2 normally varies with respiration.

8. The S_____ is an early diastolic filling sound.

9. The S3 is best heard at the cardiac apex with the _____ of the stethescope.

10. True or False: In patients over the age of 35, an S3 is considered pathologic.

11. True or False: The S3 may also be referred to as the protodiastolic gallop or ventricular gallop.

12. True or False: The S3 heart sound is associated with conditions that increase early diastolic filling.

13. The S___ is a low pitched heart sound that occurs in response to atrial contraction.

14. The S4 is best heard at the cardiac apex with the _____ of the stethescope.

15. True or False: The S4 indicates decreased ventricular compliance.

16. True or False: The S4 may also be called an atrial or presystolic gallop.

17. A loud S1 may indicate the presence of rheumatic mitral _____.

18. An atrioventricular valve opening snap is commonly associated with rheumatic _____.

19. An ejection sound or click may indicate the presence of congenital semilunar valve _____.

20. The midsystolic click may indicate the presence of mitral valve _____.

21. Fixed split S2 is associated with _____ _____ defect.

22. A pericardial _____ _____ is associated with pericarditis.

23. A pericardial _____ is associated with constrictive pericarditis.

BOARD REVIEW QUESTIONS - Section 5B

1. S1 is caused by:
    a. mitral and tricuspid valve closure
    b. mitral and tricuspid valve opening
    c. aortic and pulmonic valve closure
    d. aortic and pulmonic valve opening

2. For cardiac auscultation, the mitral area is considered to be the:
    a. lower left sternal border
    b. cardiac apex
    c. right upper sternal border
    d. left upper sternal border

3. For cardiac auscultation, the tricuspid area is considered to be the:
    a. lower left sternal border
    b. cardiac apex
    c. right upper sternal border
    d. left upper sternal border

4. S2 is caused by:
    a. mitral and tricuspid valve closure
    b. mitral and tricuspid valve opening
    c. aortic and pulmonic valve closure
    d. aortic and pulmonic valve opening

5. For cardiac auscultation, the aortic area is the:
    a. lower left sternal border
    b. cardiac apex
    c. right upper sternal border
    d. left upper sternal border

6. For cardiac auscultation, the pulmonic area is the:
    a. lower left sternal border
    b. cardiac apex
    c. right upper sternal border
    d. left upper sternal border

7. With inspiration, the interval between the two components of S2, aortic and pulmonic valve closure is:
    a. increased
    b. unchanged
    c. decreased
    d. cannot be predicted

8. The S3 occurs in:
    a. ventricular systole
    b. early ventricular diastole
    c. late ventricular diastole
    d. atrial systole

9. Another term used to describe the S3 is:
    a. presystolic gallop
    b. atrial gallop
    c. protodiastolic gallop
    d. summation gallop

10. All of the following pathologies are associated with an S3 except:
    a. aortic regurgitation
    b. mitral stenosis
    c. atrial septal defect
    d. anemia

11. The S4 occurs in response to:
    a. early ventricular diastole
    b. atrial systole
    c. ventricular diastasis
    d. ventricular systole

12. The S4 indicates:
    a. increased early diastolic filling
    b. increased ventricular contraction
    c. decreased ventricular compliance
    d. decreased atrial contraction

13. A loud S1 may indicate the presence of:
    a. aortic regurgitation
    b. mitral stenosis
    c. decreased ventricular compliance
    d. increased early diastolic filling

14. An opening snap is associated with:
    a. atrioventricular valve stenosis
    b. pulmonary regurgitation
    c. decreased ventricular compliance
    d. increased early diastolic filling

15. An ejection sound or click is associated with:
    a. mitral stenosis
    b. pulmonary regurgitation
    c. semilunar valve stenosis
    d. decreased ventricular compliance

16. The midsystolic click may indicate the presence of mitral valve:
    a. stenosis
    b. prolapse
    c. flail
    d. endocarditis

17. Fixed split S2 is associated with:
    a. atrial septal defect
    b. ventricular septal defect
    c. patent ductus arteriosus
    d. bicuspid aortic valve

18. Which of the following heart sounds is associated with pericarditis?
    a. loud S1
    b. soft S2
    c. pericardial friction rub
    d. pericardial knock

19. Which of the following heart sounds is associated with constrictive pericarditis?
    a. ejection sound
    b. midsystolic click
    c. pericardial friction rub
    d. pericardial knock

ANSWERS - Section 5B

Review practice answers

1. 1
2. apex
3. True
4. 2
5. right
6. left
7. True
8. 3
9. bell
10. True
11. True
12. True
13. 4
14. bell
15. True
16. True
17. stenosis
18. stenosis
19. stenosis
20. prolapse
21. atrial septal
22. friction rub
23. knock

Board review answers

1. a
2. b
3. a
4. c
5. c
6. d
7. a
8. b
9. c
10. b
11. b
12. c
13. b
14. a
15. c
16. b
17. a
18. c
19. d

Murmurs

A cardiac murmur is caused by turbulent blood flow moving through the heart or great vessels. Murmurs are categorized by their location, timing, intensity, configuration, pitch and quality.

Location: The mitral area is the cardiac apex. The tricuspid area is the lower left sternal border or xyphoid area. The aortic area is the right upper sternal border. The pulmonic area is the left upper sternal border.

Timing: A murmur may be systolic, diastolic or continuous. The systolic murmur can be characterized as early, mid, late or holosystolic (pansystolic). The diastolic murmur may be described as early or mid to late.

Intensity: A murmur may be graded on a scale from I to VI. A grade I murmur is barely audible; grade II is faintly heard; grade III is moderately loud; grade IV is loud; grade V is very loud and grade VI is loud with a thrill and can be heard with the stethescope lifted off the surface of the chest.

Configuration: A murmur may be described by its change in intensity. A crescendo murmur begins softly and becomes louder. A decrescendo murmur begins loud and becomes softer. A crescendo-decrescendo murmur begins softly, becomes louder, and then decreases in intensity. A decrescendo-crescendo murmur begins loudly, becomes softer, then builds to the original intensity.

Pitch: The pitch of a murmur is determined by blood flow velocity. A high pitched murmur is best heard with the diaphragm. A low pitched murmur is best heard with the bell of the stethescope. A murmur that is heard best with both the diaphragm and bell of the stethescope is a medium pitch murmur.

Quality: A murmur's quality may be described as blowing, rumbling, harsh, dull or rasping.

Early systolic murmurs: Early systolic murmurs begin with the first heart sound and end in midsystole. The common causes of early systolic murmurs include:
Small ventricular septal defect,
A large ventricular septal defect with pulmonary hypertension
Severe acute mitral or tricuspid regurgitation.

Systolic ejection murmurs: Systolic ejection murmurs begin after the semilunar valves open. The causes include:
Valvular aortic or pulmonic stenosis
Dilatation of the aorta or pulmonary artery
Increased rate of ejection (heart block, fever, anemia, exercise, thyrotoxicosis, and sometimes is heard in normal individuals).

Pansystolic (holosystolic) murmurs: Pansystolic (holosystolic) murmurs are present when there is flow between two chambers that have widely different pressures throughout systole, such as the left ventricle and the left atrium in mitral regurgitation. The most common causes include:
Mitral regurgitation or tricuspid regurgitation
Ventricular septal defects
Aortopulmonary shunts.

Late systolic murmurs: Late systolic murmurs are faint or moderately loud high-pitched apical murmurs that start well after ejection and do not mask either normal heart sound. The most common causes include:

Papillary muscle dysfunction in patients with myocardial ischemia or infarction.

Late systolic murmurs following midsystolic clicks are associated with late systolic mitral regurgitation caused by prolapse of the mitral valve.

Early diastolic murmurs: Early diastolic murmurs begin immediately after the second heart sound. The most common cause is:

Aortic valve regurgitation
Pulmonic valve regurgitation

Mid-diastolic and late diastolic murmurs: Mid-diastolic and late diastolic murmurs are produced by the forward flow of blood through the atrioventricular valves. The murmur is low pitched and rumbling in quality. The causes include:

Mitral valve stenosis
Tricuspid valve stenosis
Left atrial myxoma (which may simulate a "stenotic" valve)
Mitral regurgitation (increased flow)
Large left-to-right shunts (increased flow).

Continuous murmurs: Continuous murmurs may result from blood flow constantly moving from a high-pressure area to a low-pressure area. The causes include:

Patent ductus arteriosus
Systemic arteriovenous fistula
Coronary artery from the pulmonary artery
Communications between the sinus of Valsalva and the right side of the heart.

Response to physiologic maneuvers

Valsalva Maneuvers: Most murmurs decrease during the strain phase of the Valsalva maneuver except hypertrophic obstructive cardiomyopathy and mitral valve prolapse.

Isometric Handgrip: Sustained isometric handgrip increases peripheral resistance, blood pressure, heart rate and cardiac output. The handgrip increases the left heart murmurs of mitral regurgitation, aortic regurgitation and ventricular septal defect. The murmurs of semilunar valve stenosis and hypertrophic obstructive cardiomyopathy will be reduced with sustained isometric handgrip.

Amyl Nitrite: Amyl nitrite is a fast acting vasodilator. The inhalation of amyl nitrite will initially decrease venous return and blood pressure. It will augment left ventricular outflow tract obstruction murmurs such as hypertrophic obstructive cardiomyopathy. Mitral valve prolapse may be enhanced with amyl nitrite inhalation. Amyl nitrite will decrease the murmurs of aortic regurgitation, mitral regurgitation and ventricular septal defect. The forward flow murmurs such as mitral valve stenosis increase with the administration of amyl nitrite.

192

DISEASE/MURMUR CONFIGURATION	MURMER CHARACTERISTICS

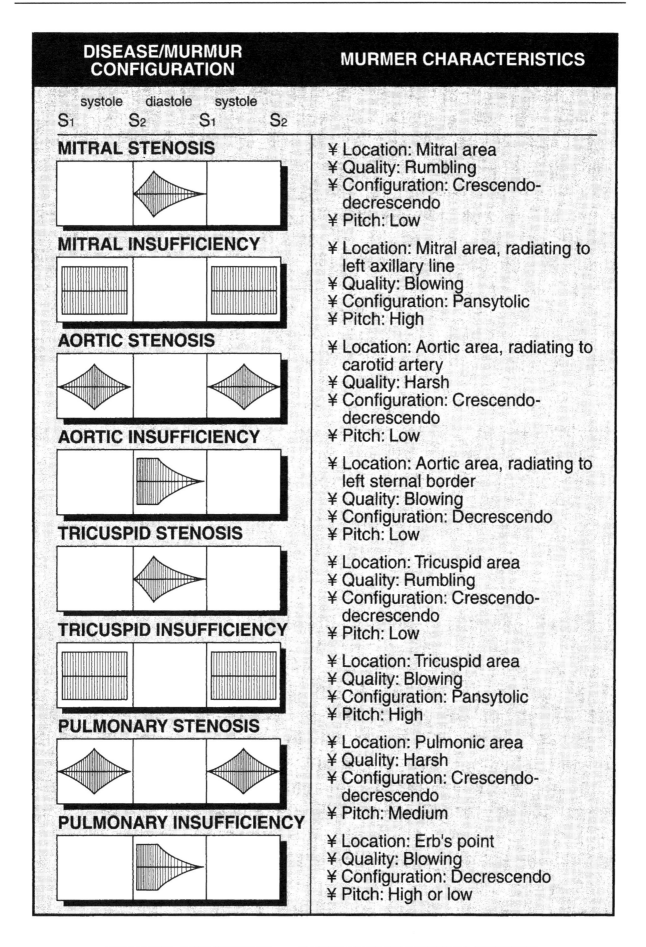

MITRAL STENOSIS	¥ Location: Mitral area ¥ Quality: Rumbling ¥ Configuration: Crescendo-decrescendo ¥ Pitch: Low
MITRAL INSUFFICIENCY	¥ Location: Mitral area, radiating to left axillary line ¥ Quality: Blowing ¥ Configuration: Pansytolic ¥ Pitch: High
AORTIC STENOSIS	¥ Location: Aortic area, radiating to carotid artery ¥ Quality: Harsh ¥ Configuration: Crescendo-decrescendo ¥ Pitch: Low
AORTIC INSUFFICIENCY	¥ Location: Aortic area, radiating to left sternal border ¥ Quality: Blowing ¥ Configuration: Decrescendo ¥ Pitch: Low
TRICUSPID STENOSIS	¥ Location: Tricuspid area ¥ Quality: Rumbling ¥ Configuration: Crescendo-decrescendo ¥ Pitch: Low
TRICUSPID INSUFFICIENCY	¥ Location: Tricuspid area ¥ Quality: Blowing ¥ Configuration: Pansytolic ¥ Pitch: High
PULMONARY STENOSIS	¥ Location: Pulmonic area ¥ Quality: Harsh ¥ Configuration: Crescendo-decrescendo ¥ Pitch: Medium
PULMONARY INSUFFICIENCY	¥ Location: Erb's point ¥ Quality: Blowing ¥ Configuration: Decrescendo ¥ Pitch: High or low

systole   diastole   systole
S₁   S₂   S₁   S₂

REVIEW PRACTICE - Section 5B

1. A _____ is caused by turbulent blood flow moving through the heart or great vessels.

2. For cardiac auscultation, the mitral area is the cardiac _____.

3. For cardiac auscultation, the tricuspid area is the lower _____ sternal border or _____ area.

4. For cardiac auscultation, the aortic area is the _____ upper sternal border.

5. For cardiac auscultation, the pulmonic area is the _____ upper sternal border.

6. A cardiac murmur may occur in _____, _____ or _____.

7. True or False: The systolic murmur may be characterized as early, mid, late or holosytolic (pansystolic).

8. The diastolic murmur may be described as _____ or mid to late.

9. A grade _____ murmur is barely audible.

10. A grade _____ murmur is faintly heard.

11. A grade _____ murmur is moderately loud.

12. A grade _____ murmur is loud.

13. A grade _____ murmur is very loud.

14. A grade _____ murmur is loud with a thrill and may be heard with the stethescope lifted off the chest wall.

15. True or False: A grade III murmur or higher is considered a clinically significant murmur.

16. A _____ murmur begins softly and becomes louder.

17. A _____ murmur begins loud and becomes softer.

18. A _____-_____ murmur begins softly, becomes louder, and then decreases in intensity.

19. A _____-_____ murmur begins loud, becomes softer, then increases in intensity.

20. The _____ of a murmur is determined by blood flow velocity.

21. A low pitched murmur is best heard with the _____ of the stethescope.

22. A high pitched murmur is best heard with the _____ of the stethescope.

23. A murmur that is heard equally well with both the diaphragm and bell of the stethescope is a _____ pitched murmur.

24. True or False: The quality of a murmur may be decribed as blowing, rumbling, harsh, dull or rasping.

25. The _____ systolic murmur begins with the first heart sound and ends in midsystole.

CHAPTER 5 (UNIT FIVE) - CARDIAC EVALUATION METHODS

26. Check the following if a possible cause of an early systolic murmur:
    _____small ventricular septal defect
    _____large ventricular septal defect with pulmonary hypertension
    _____severe acute mitral regurgitation

27. The systolic _____ murmur begins after the semilunar valves open.

28. Check the following if a possible cause of a systolic ejection murmur:
    _____valvular aortic/pulmonic stenosis
    _____aortic/pulmonary artery dilatation
    _____increased rate of ejection

29. The _____ or _____ murmur occurs when there is flow between two chambers that have widely different pressures throughout systole.

30. Check the following if a possible cause of a pansystolic murmur:
    _____mitral/tricuspid regurgitation
    _____ventricular septal defect
    _____aortopulmonary shunts

31. The _____ systolic murmur starts well after ejection.

32. Check the following if a possible cause of a late systolic murmur:
    _____ papillary muscle dysfunction
    _____ mitral valve prolapse

33. The _____ diastolic murmur begins immediately after the second heart sound.

34. The _____-diastolic and _____ diastolic murmurs are produced by forward flow of blood through the atrioventricular valve.

35. Check the following if a possible cause of a mid-diastolic or late diastolic murmur:
    _____mitral/tricuspid stenosis
    _____left atrial myxoma
    _____mitral regurgitation
    _____large left-to-right shunts

36. The _____ murmur may result from blood flow constantly from a high pressure area to a low pressure area.

37. Check the following if a possible cause of a continuous murmur:
    _____patent ductus arteriosus
    _____systemic atreriovenous fistula
    _____coronary artery orginating from the pulmonary artery
    _____ruptured sinus of Valsalva

38. True or False: Most murmurs increase in intensity except hypertrophic obstructive cardiomyopathy and mitral valve prolapse during the strain phase of the Valsalva maneuver.

39. True or False: The isometric handgrip will reduce the murmur of valvular aortic stenosis and hypertrophic obstructive cardiomyopathy.

40. True or False: The isometric handgrip will increase the intensity of the murmur of mitral regurgitation.

41. True or False: Amyl nitrite will increase the intensity of the mitral stenosis murmur.

42. True or False: Amyl nitrite will increase the intensity of aortic regurgitation and pulmonic regurgitation murmurs.

43. Amyl nitrite will increase?/decrease? the murmur of hypertrophic obstructive cardiomyopathy.

44. True or False: Amyl nitrite will enhance mitral valve prolapse.

CHAPTER 5 (UNIT FIVE) - CARDIAC EVALUATION METHODS

BOARD REVIEW QUESTIONS - Section 5B

1. Which of the following is incorrect when describing the auscultation areas for the cardiac valves?
   a. aortic: right upper sternal border
   b. pulmonic: left upper sternal border
   c. mitral: lower left sternal border
   d. tricuspid: xyphoid area

2. A grade I murmur is a murmur that is:
   a. loud
   b. moderately loud
   c. faintly heard
   d. barely heard

3. A grade II murmur is a murmur that is:
   a. barely heard
   b. loud
   c. moderately loud
   d. faintly heard

4. A grade III murmur is a murmur that is:
   a. barely heard
   b. faintly heard
   c. moderately loud
   d. loud

5. A grade IV murmur is a murmur that is:
   a. barely heard
   b. faintly heard
   c. moderately loud
   d. loud

6. A grade V murmur is a murmur that is:
   a. moderately loud
   b. loud
   c. very loud
   d. loud with a thrill

7. A grade VI murmur is a murmur that is:
   a. moderately loud
   b. loud
   c. very loud
   d. loud with a thrill

8. A _____ murmur is one that begins softly and becomes louder.
    a. crescendo
    b. decrescendo
    c. crescendo-decrescendo
    d. decrescendo-crescendo

9. A _____ murmur is a murmur that begins loud and becomes softer.
    a. crescendo
    b. decrescendo
    c. crescendo-decrescendo
    d. decrescendo-crescendo

10. A _____ murmur begins softly, becomes louder, and then decreases in loudness.
    a. decrescendo-crescendo
    b. crescendo-decrescendo
    c. decrescendo
    d. crescendo

11. A _____ murmur begins loud, becomes softer, and then increases in loudness.
    a. decrescendo-crescendo
    b. crescendo-decrescendo
    c. crescendo
    d. decrescendo

12. A low pitched murmur is best heard with the stethescope's:
    a. bell
    b. diaphragm
    c. both bell and diaphragm
    d. varies

13. A medium pitched murmur is best heard with the stethescope's:
    a. bell
    b. diaphragm
    c. both bell and diaphragm
    d. varies

14. A high pitched murmur is best heard with the stethescope's:
    a. bell
    b. diaphragm
    c. bell and diaphragm
    d. varies

15. Which of the following murmurs begin with the first heart sound and end in midsystole?
    a. early systolic
    b. systolic ejection
    c. holosystolic
    d. late systolic

16. All of the following are possible causes of early systolic murmurs except:
    a. valvular aortic stenosis
    b. small ventricular septal defect
    c. large ventricular septal defect with pulmonary hypertension
    d. severe acute mitral/tricuspid regurgitation

17. Which of the following murmurs begins after the semilunar valves open?
    a. early systolic
    b. systolic ejection
    c. holosystolic
    d. late systolic

18. All of the following are associated with a systolic ejection murmur except:
    a. valvular aortic/pulmonic stenosis
    b. aortic/pulmonic dilatation
    c. anemia
    d. ventricular septal defect

19. Which of the following murmurs is present when there is flow between two chambers that have widely different pressures throughout systole?
    a. early systolic
    b. systolic ejection
    c. pansystolic
    d. late systolic

20. All of the following are considered to be associated with a pansystolic murmur except:
    a. mitral/tricuspid regurgitation
    b. ventricular septal defect
    c. aortopulmonary shunts
    d. mitral valve prolapse

21. Which of the following murmurs start well after ejection?
    a. early systolic ejection
    b. late systolic
    c. holosystolic
    d. systolic ejection

22. All of the following are associated with a late systolic murmur except:
    a. papillary muscle dysfunction
    b. myocardial ischemia/infraction
    c. valvular pulmonic stenosis
    d. mitral valve prolapse

23. Which of the following murmurs begins immediately after the second heart sound?
    a. early diastolic
    b. mid-diastolic
    c. late diastolic
    d. continuous

24. Which of the following is most likely to cause an early diastolic murmur?
    a. aortic valve regurgitation
    b. mitral valve prolapse
    c. patent ductus arteriosus
    d. ventricular septal defect

25. Which of the following murmurs is caused by forward flow across an atrioventricular valve?
    a. early diastolic
    b. mid-diastolic
    c. continuous
    d. early systolic

26. All of the following are associated with a mid-diastolic or late diastolic murmur except:
    a. mitral/tricuspid stenosis
    b. left atrial myxoma
    c. mitral/tricuspid regurgitation
    d. aortic regurgitation

27. Which of the following murmurs may result from blood flow constantly moving from a high pressure to a low pressure area?
    a. early diastolic
    b. mid-diastolic
    c. late diastolic
    d. continuous

28. All of the following are associated with a continuous murmur except:
    a. patent ductus arteriosus
    b. systemic arteriovenous fistula
    c. severe mitral regurgitation
    d. coronary artery from the pulmonary artery

29. Which effect will the strain phase of the Valsalva maneuver have on venous return?
    a. increase
    b. decrease
    c. varies
    d. cannot be predicted

30. All of the following murmurs will decrease in intensity during the strain phase of the Valsalva maneuver except:
    a. valvular aortic stenosis
    b. mitral stenosis
    c. hypertrophic obstructive cardiomyopathy
    d. tricuspid regurgitation

31. What effect will the isometric handgrip have on mitral regurgitation?
    a. increase
    b. decrease
    c. varies
    d. cannot be predicted

32. What effect will the isometric handgrip have on valvular aortic stenosis?
    a. increase
    b. decrease
    c. varies
    d. cannot be predicted

33. What effect will the inhalation of amyl nitrite have on a ventricular septal defect murmur?
    a. increase
    b. decrease
    c. varies
    d. cannot be predicted

34. What effect will the inhalation of amyl nitrite have on left heart regurgitant murmurs?
    a. increase
    b. decrease
    c. varies
    d. cannot be predicted

35. What effect will the inhalation of amyl nitrite have on the murmur of hypertrophic obstructive cardiomyopathy?
    a. increase
    b. decrease
    c. varies
    d. cannot be predicted

36. What effect will the inhalation of amyl nitrite have on mitral valve prolapse?
    a. increase
    b. decrease
    c. varies
    d. cannot be predicted

ANSWERS - Section 5B

Review practice answers

1. murmur
2. apex
3. left, xyphoid
4. right
5. left
6. diastole, systole, continuous
7. True
8. early
9. I
10. II
11. III
12. IV
13. V
14. VI
15. True
16. crescendo
17. decrescendo
18. crescendo-decrescendo
19. decrescendo-crescendo
20. pitch
21. bell
22. diaphragm
23. medium
24. True
25. early
26. all
27. ejection
28. all
29. pansystolic, holosystolic
30. all
31. late
32. all
33. early
34. mid, late
35. all
36. continuous
37. all
38. False
39. True
40. True

41. True
42. False
43. increase
44. True

Board review answers

1. c
2. d
3. d
4. c
5. d
6. c
7. d
8. a
9. b
10. b
11. a
12. a
13. c
14. b
15. a
16. a
17. b
18. d
19. c
20. d
21. b
22. c
23. a
24. a
25. b
26. d
27. d
28. c
29. b
30. c
31. a
32. b
33. b
34. b
35. a
36. a

SECTION 5C
Electrocardiography (EKG)

1. BASIC PRINCIPLES AND WAVEFORMS

The electrocardiogram presents a visible record of the heart's electrical activity by tracing the activity on a continuously moving strip of paper. The normal electrocardiogram consists of three waves.

Electrocardiogram waves

P wave: A small, positive deflection caused by atrial depolarization and relates to atrial systole.

QRS complex: A triphasic waveform which coincides with ventricular depolarization and ventricular contraction. The Q wave is the first negative deflection after the P wave. The R wave is a tall, spiked shaped positive deflection. The S wave is a negative deflection following the R wave.

T wave: A positive deflection that is related to ventricular repolarization.

The normal electrical pathway

The electrical impulse originates from the normal physiologic pacemaker, the sinoatrial node. The impulse spreads through the atria via the internodal pathways to the atrioventricular (AV) node. After a brief delay, the impulse continues through the bundle of His, the right and left bundle branches, Purkinje fibers and finally activates the ventricular muscle cells. Both the SA and AV nodes are innervated by the sympathetic nervous system, which increases the heart rate and the parasympathetic (vagus nerve) nervous system which decreases the heart rate.

The SA node fires electrical impulses at a rate of 60-100 times per minute, AV junctional tissue at 40-60 and the Purkinje fibers at 20-40.

Normal sinus rhythm

The rate is regular and the heart rate is between 60-100 beats per minute. The P waves and QRS complexes are uniform and there is a P wave for each QRS complex.

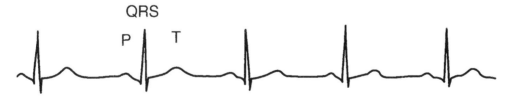

2. COMMON ABNORMALITIES

Sinus bradycardia: All complexes are normal but the heart rate is below 60 beats per minute.

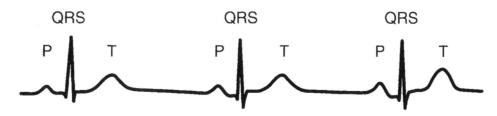

CHAPTER 5 (UNIT FIVE) - CARDIAC EVALUATION METHODS

Sinus tachycardia: All the complexes are normal but the heart rate is above 100 beats per minute.

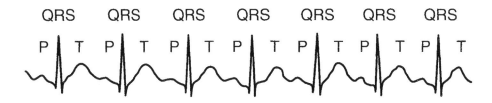

Sinus arrhythmia: All complexes are normal but the rate increases and decreases with respiration.

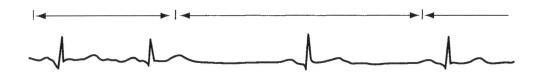

Sinus pause or sinus arrest: The SA node fails to send out an impulse for a period of time.

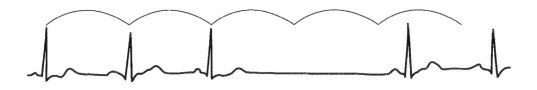

Premature atrial contraction (PAC): A PAC occurs when an atrial pacemaker other than the SA node discharges an electrical impulse, which creates an abnormal P wave. Normal sinus rhythm is interrupted although heart rate and QRS complexes are uniform. A pause usually follows the PAC.

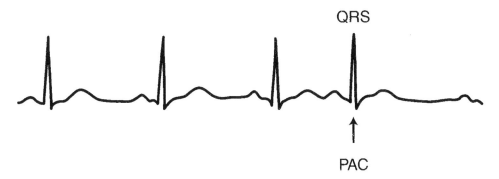

Left atrial enlargement: Left atrial enlargement is best detected using lead V1 with the criteria being a biphasic P wave with a wide, deep negative component that is at least one box wide and one box deep.

Right atrial enlargement: A P wave amplitude of greater than 2.5 mm in leads II, III and AVF.

CHAPTER 5 (UNIT FIVE) - CARDIAC EVALUATION METHODS

Atrial flutter: With atrial flutter, there is rapid, regular fluttering of the atrium at a rate of between 250 and 350 beats per minute. The P waves are sawtooth in appearance. A QRS complex does not follow each P wave.

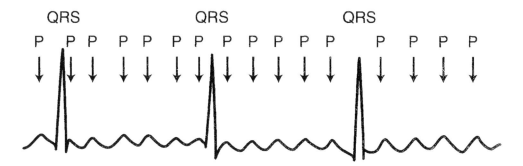

Atrial fibrillation: Atrial fibrillation is caused by multiple atrial ectopic foci. There is no well defined P wave, the QRS complex is normal although the ventricular rate is irregular. The atrial rate ranges from 400 to 700 impulses per minute.

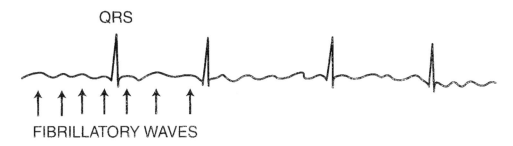

Left ventricular hypertrophy: The sum of the S wave depth in V1 or V2 and the R wave height in V5 or V6 greater than 35 mm.

Right ventricular hypertrophy: A dominant R wave in lead V1 greater than 7 mm in height.

Premature ventricular contraction (PVC): A PVC originates from an ectopic foci in the ventricle. PVC's occur early in the cycle, the QRS complex is wide and distorted and may be followed by a compensatory pause. A P wave does not usually precede a PVC. Unifocal PVC's originate from the same location and have the same configuration. Multifocal PVC's originate from multiple sites and therefore have different shapes. Bigeminy is the repeating pattern of two beats with PVC's and normal beats alternating. Trigeminy is a repeating pattern of three beats with the ratio of PVC's to normal beats 2:1.

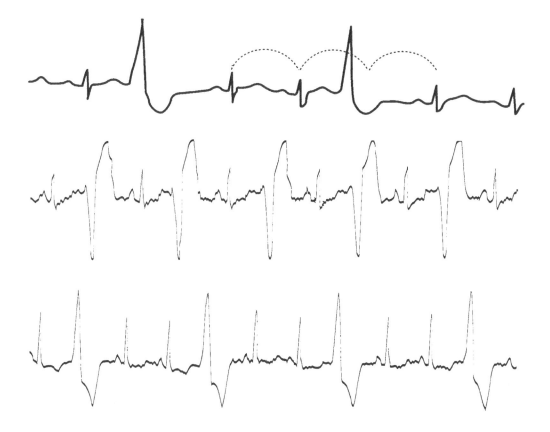

Ventricular tachycardia: Consecutive PVC's (three or more) with a heart rate of between 150 to 200 beats per minute.

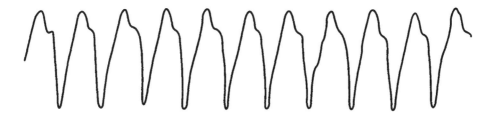

Ventricular fibrillation: Since there are numerous ventricular ectopic foci firing simultaneously, there is a complete absence of a heart rhythm. There is complete distortion and irregularity demonstrated on the electrocardiogram.

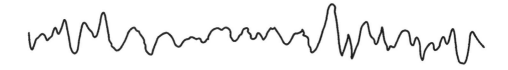

Left bundle branch block: A QRS wave duration greater than 0.12 seconds and large, broad, notched or slurred R waves in leads I, AVL, V5 and/or V6.

Right bundle branch block: A QRS duration of greater than 0.12 seconds and a triphasic QRS complex (RSR') in leads V1 - V3.

First degree atrioventricular (AV) block: The PR interval is abnormally increased to over 0.20 seconds. All P waves are followed by a QRS complex.

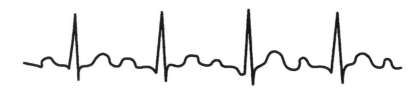

CHAPTER 5 (UNIT FIVE) - CARDIAC EVALUATION METHODS

Second degree atrioventricular block: There are two classifications of this condition. In Mobitz I (Wenckebach), there is progressive lengthening of the PR interval until a beat is blocked and then the cycle is repeated. In Mobitz II, some beats are conducted while others are not.

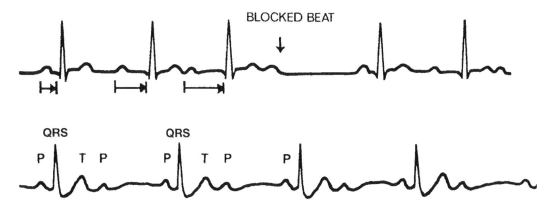

Third degree AV block: Also referred to as complete heart block since no atrial impulses will activate the ventricles. The P waves and the QRS complexes occur indepedent of each other.

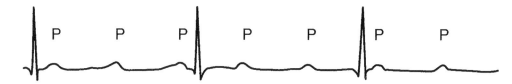

Wolff-Parkinson-White (WPW): A prexcitation syndrome where the atrial impulse is transmitted directly to the ventricles via shortcut conduction pathways. A short PR interval (less than 0.12 seconds), a slurred upstroke of the QRS complex (delta wave) and a wide QRS complex (greater than 0.12 seconds) indicates the presence of WPW. WPW is associated with Ebstein's anomaly.

Myocardial ischemia: The classic electrocardiogram finding for myocardial ischemia during an exercise stress test is ST segment depression.

Myocardial infarction: A new myocardial infarction is characterized by ST segment elevation and T wave inversion. An abnormal Q wave (greater than 0.04 seconds wide or greater in depth than one-third the height of the QRS complex) is indicative of an old infarction. The electrocardiogram may be used to predict the location of the infarction. An inferior wall infarction will demonstrate changes in leads II, III and AVF. An antero-septal infarction will demonstrate changes in leads V1-V2. An anterior wall infarction will cause changes in leads V3-V4. A lateral wall infarction will demonstrate changes in leads I, AVL and/or V5-V6. ST segment elevation which persists may indicate the formation of a ventricular aneurysm.

Acute Pericarditis: The acute phase of pericarditis will cause ST segment elevation in the precordial leads especially leads V5-V6.

CHAPTER 5 (UNIT FIVE) - CARDIAC EVALUATION METHODS

Artificial pacemaker: The pacemaker delivers an electrical impulse to the heart and this is marked on the electrocardiogram as a spike. The spike will be seen in front of each QRS complex if the pacemaker electrode rests in the ventricle. The spike will appear in front of each P wave if the electrode rests in the atrium. If there is a pacemaker electrode in the atrium and ventricle a pacemaker spike will appear in front of each P wave and QRS complex.

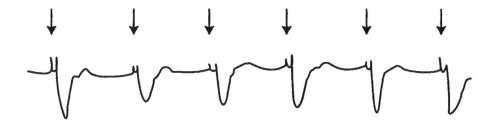

REVIEW PRACTICE - Section 5C

1. The _____ presents a visible record of the heart's electrical activity.

2. True or False: The term electrocardiogram may be abbreviated as EKG or ECG.

3. True or False: The normal electrocardiogram consists of three waves.

4. The _____ wave represents atrial depolarization and atrial systole.

5. The _____ complex is a triphasic wave that represents ventricular depolarization and ventricular systole.

6. The _____ wave is a positive deflection representing ventricular repolarization.

7. The electrical impulse orginates in the _____ atrial node travels through the internodal pathways to the _____ node through the bundle of _____, to the _____ and _____ bundle branches and finally to the _____ fibers.

8. The SA node normally emits electrical impulses at a rate of between _____ to _____ times per minute.

9. The EKG strip shown below is demonstrating _____ sinus rhythm.

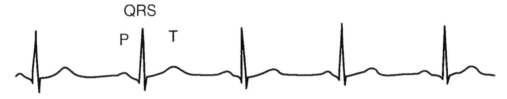

10. The EKG strip shown below is demonstrating sinus _____.

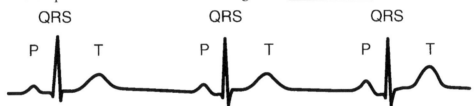

11. The EKG strip shown below is demonstrating sinus _____.

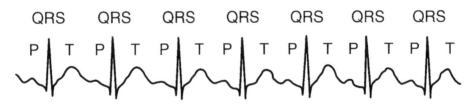

12. The EKG strip shown below is demonstrating sinus _____.

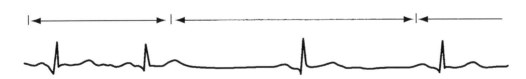

13. The EKG strip shown below is demonstrating sinus _____ or sinus _____.

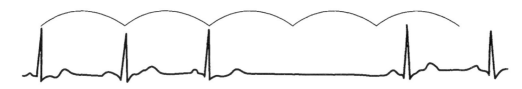

14. The EKG strip shown below is demonstrating premature _____ contractions.

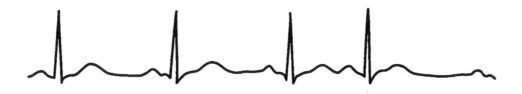

15. The EKG strip shown below is demonstrating atrial _____.

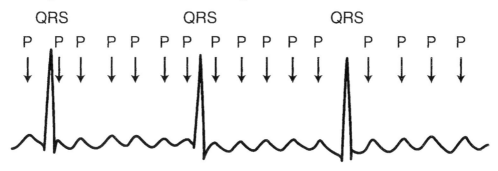

16. The EKG strip shown below is demonstrating atrial _____.

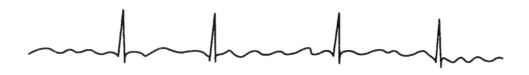

17. The EKG strip shown below is demonstrating premature _____ contractions.

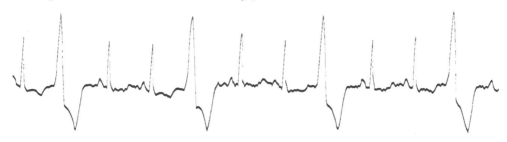

18. The EKG strip shown below is demonstrating ventricular _____.

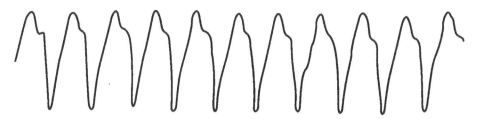

19. The EKG strip shown below is demonstrating ventricular _____.

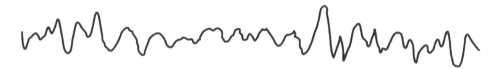

20. The EKG strip shown below is demonstrating _____ degree AV block.

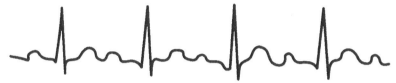

21. The EKG strip shown below is demonstrating _____ degree AV block. This is also referred to as _____

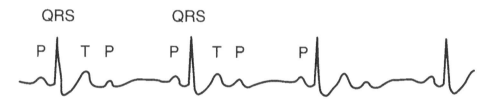

22. The EKG strip shown below is demonstrating _____ degree AV block.

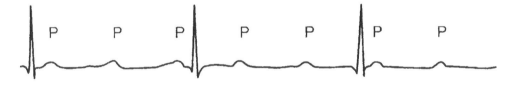

23. True or False: ST segmant elevation throughout the precordial leads especially in leads V5-V6 may indicate the presence of acute pericarditis.

24. The EKG strip shown below is demonstrating an artificial _____.

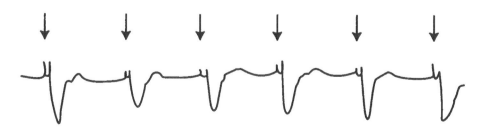

CHAPTER 5 (UNIT FIVE) - CARDIAC EVALUATION METHODS

BOARD REVIEW QUESTIONS - Section 5C

1. The EKG strip shown below is demonstrating:
   a. normal sinus ryhthm
   b. sinus bradycardia
   c. sinus tachycardia
   d. sinus arrest

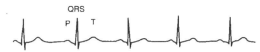

2. The EKG strip shown below is demonstrating:
   a. normal sinus ryhthm
   b. sinus bradycardia
   c. sinus tachycardia
   d. sinus arrest

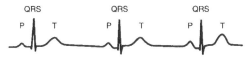

3. The EKG strip shown below is demonstrating:
   a. normal sinus rhythm
   b. sinus bradycardia
   c. sinus tachycardia
   d. sinus arrest

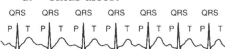

4. The EKG strip shown below is demonstrating:
   a. normal sinus ryhthm
   b. sinus tachycardia
   c. sinus bradycardia
   d. sinus arrythmia

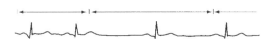

5. The EKG strip shown below is demonstrating:
   a. sinus bradycardia
   b. sinus tachycardia
   c. sinus arrythmia
   d. sinus pause

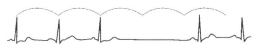

6. The EKG strip shown below is demonstrating:
    a. premature atrial contraction
    b. atrial flutter
    c. atrial fibrillation
    d. premature ventricular contraction

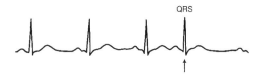

7. The EKG strip shown below is demonstrating:
    a. premature atrial contractions
    b. atrial flutter
    c. atrial fibrillation
    d. premature ventricular contractions

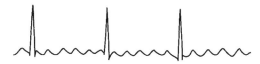

8. The EKG strip shown below is demonstrating:
    a. premature atrial contractions
    b. atrial flutter
    c. atrial fibrillation
    d. premature ventricular contractions

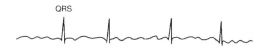

9. The EKG strip shown below is demonstrating:
    a. premature atrial contractions
    b. atrial flutter
    c. atrial fibrillation
    d. premature ventricular contractions

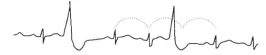

10. The EKG strip shown below is demonstrating:
    a. ventricular tachycardia
    b. ventricular fibrillation
    c. first degree AV block
    d. second degree AV block

11. The EKG strip shown below is demonstrating:
    a. ventricular tachycardia
    b. ventricular fibrillation
    c. first degree AV block
    d. second degree AV block

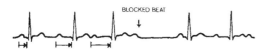

12. The EKG strip shown below is demonstrating:
    a. ventricular tachycardia
    b. ventricular fibrillation
    c. first degree AV block
    d. second degree AV block

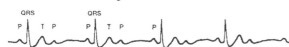

13. The EKG strip shown below is demonstrating:
    a. ventricular tachycardia
    b. ventricular fibrillation
    c. first degree AV block
    d. second degree AV block

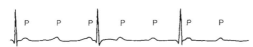

14. The EKG strip shown below is demonstrating:
    a. first degree AV block
    b. second degree AV block
    c. third degree AV block
    d. artificial pacemaker

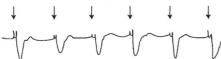

15. The EKG strip shown below is demonstrating:
    a. first degree AV block
    b. second degree AV block
    c. third degree AV block
    d. Wolff-Parkinson-White syndrome

16. The EKG strip shown below is demonstrating:
    a. first degree AV block
    b. Mobitz I
    c. Wenckebach
    d. artificial pacemaker

ANSWERS - Section 5C

Review practice answers

1. electrocardiogram
2. True
3. True
4. P
5. QRS
6. T
7. sino, atrioventricular, His, right, left, Purkinje
8. 60, 100
9. normal
10. bradycardia
11. tachycardia
12. arrhythmia
13 pause, arrest
14. atrial
15. flutter
16. fibrillation
17. ventricular
18. tachycardia
19. fibrillation
20. first
21. second, Mobitz
22. third
23. True
24. pacemaker

Board review answers

1. a
2. b
3. c
4. d
5. d
6. a
7. b
8. c
9. d
10. a
11. b
12. c
13. d
14. c
15. c
16. d

3. EXERCISE AND PHARMACOLOGIC STRESS TESTING

Exercise stress testing is used to evaluate the cardiovascular response to exercise. An electrocardiogram is an integral component of the stress test being utilized to detect EKG changes due to myocardial ischemia.

Theory: An increase in myocardial oxygen demand during exercise must be met by an increase in coronary artery blood flow or ischemia will result.

Indications: Chest pain
Assessment of cardiovascular fitness
Evaluation of therapy for arrhythmias and angina
Evaluation of the asymptomatic patient with risk factors

Interpretation: A stress test may be considered positive for coronary artery disease if one or more of the following is present during the stress test examination:
ST segment depression
Chest pain
Hypotension
Failure of blood pressure to rise
Arrhythmias
ST segment elevation
R wave changes
Decreased duration of exercise

Pharmacological agents

Dobutamine: A potent positive inotrope and chronotrope which will increase myocardial oxygen consumption.

Dipyridamole (Persantine): A phosphodiesterase inhibitor which dilates the coronary arteries and induces a hypoperfusion in myocardium fed by stenotic coronary arteries.

Adenosine: A potent coronary vasodilator which may induce a hypoperfusion in myocardium fed by stenotic coronary arteries.

REVIEW PRACTICE - Section 5C

1. _____ stress testing is used to evaluate the cardiovascular response to exercise.

2. True or False: An increase in myocardial oxygen demand during exercise must be met by an increase in coronary blood flow or ischemia will result.

3. Check the following if a possible indication for stress test exam:

   _____chest pain

   _____assessment of cardiovascular fitness

   _____evaluation of therapy for arryhthmias/angina

   _____evaluation of the asymptomatic patient with risk factors

4. Check the following if a possible indication that a stress test may be considered positive for coronary artery disease:

   _____ST segment depression

   _____chest pain

   _____hypotension

   _____abnormal blood pressure response

   _____arryhthmias

   _____ST segment elevation

   _____R wave changes

   _____Decrease duration of exercise

5. _____ is a potent positive inotrope and chronotrope that will increase myocardial oxygen consumption.

6. _____ dilates the coronary arteries and induces a hypoperfusion in myocardium fed by stenotic coronary arteries.

7. _____ is a potent coronary artery vasodilator which may induce a hypoperfusion in myocardium fed by stenotic coronary arteries.

BOARD REVIEW QUESTIONS - Section 5C

1. Which of the following is used to evaluate the cardiovascular response to exercise?
   a. exercise stress test
   b. electroencephalogram
   c. echocardiography
   d. auscultation

2. All of the following are indications for an exercise stress test except:
   a. chest pain
   b. arryhthmias
   c. valvular aortic stenosis
   d. assessment of cardiovascular fitness

3. Which of the following is the most reliable indicator of myocardial ischemia during a exercise stress test examination?
   a. ST segment depression
   b. hypotension
   c. decrease in R wave voltage
   d. arryhthmias

4. Which of the following is a positive inotrope and positive chronotrope?
   a. dipyridamole
   b. Persantine
   c. adenosine
   d. dobutamine

5. All of the following may induce myocardial ischemia via dilatation of the coronary arteries except:
   a. dipyridamole
   b. Persantine
   c. adenosine
   d. dobutamine

ANSWERS - Section 5C

Review practice answers

1. exercise
2. True
3. all
4. all
5. dobutamine
6. dipyridamole (Persantine)
7. adenosine

Board review answers

1. a
2. c
3. a
4. d
5. d

Section 5D
Phonocardiography

Phonocardiography is a graphic recording of heart sounds and murmurs.

A phonocardiographic examination may also include pulse tracings of the carotid and jugular as well as an apexcardiogram.

How Acquired: Microphones with transducers are placed in various locations of the chest wall to detect normal and abnormal heart sounds.

Common Cardiac Diseases/Pattern Recognition

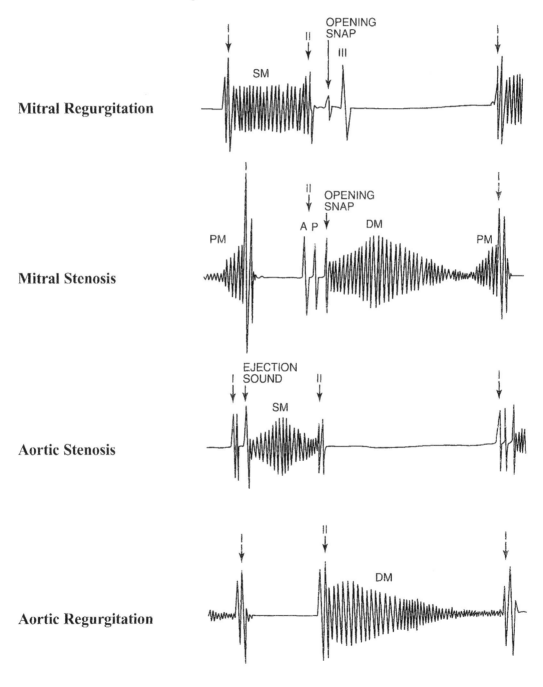

REVIEW PRACTICE - Section 5D

1. A _____ is a graphic recording of heart sounds and murmurs.

2. True or False: A phonocardiographic examination may include pulse tracings of the carotid artery and internal jugular vein and an apexcardiogram.

3. True or False: The phonocardiogram may be obtained by placing special transducers on the chest wall to detect heart sounds and murmurs.

4. The phonocardiogram shown below is _____ regurgitation.

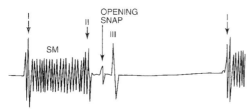

5. The phonocardiogram shown below is:_____ stenosis.

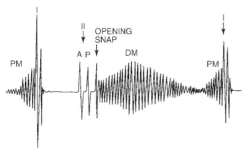

6. The phonocardiogram shown below is _____ stenosis.

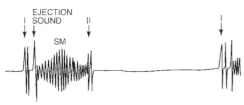

7. The phonocardiogram shown below is _____ regurgitation.

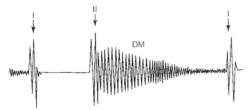

BOARD REVIEW QUESTIONS - Section 5D

1. A graphic recording of heart sounds and murmurs is the:
   a. electrocardiogram
   b. phonocardiogram
   c. echocardiogram
   d. electroencephalogram

2. All of the following may be performed during a phonocardiographic examination except:
   a. carotid pulse tracing
   b. jugular pulse tracing
   c. apexcardiogram
   d. atrial pressure tracing

3. The phonocardiogram shown below is:
   a. normal
   b. mitral stenosis
   c. mitral regurgitation
   d. mitral valve prolapse

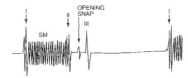

4. The phonocardiogram shown below is:
   a. normal
   b. mitral stenosis
   c. aortic stenosis
   d. aortic regurgitation

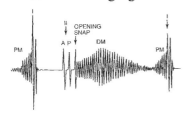

5. The phonocardiogram shown below is:
   a. normal
   b. mitral stenosis
   c. aortic stenosis
   d. aortic regurgitation

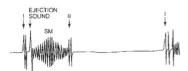

6. The phonocardiogram shown below is:
   a. normal
   b. mitral stenosis
   c. aortic stenosis
   d. aortic regurgitation

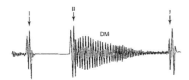

ANSWERS - Section 5D

Review practice answers

1. phonocardiogram
2. True
3. True
4. mitral
5. mitral
6. aortic
7. aortic

Board review answers

1. b
2. d
3. c
4. b
5. c
6. d

SECTION 5E
Cardiac Catheterization

1. BASIC CONCEPTS OF HEMODYNAMIC RECORDINGS

Cardiac catheterization is an invasive procedure used to visualize cardiac chambers and the coronary arterial system by introducing a catheter into the heart and great vessels. A routine cardiac catheterization usually includes a right heart and left heart catheterization and coronary arteriography.

The objectives of a cardiac catheterization include:
    To provide intracardiac pressures/oxygen saturations
    To assess ventricular function (global, segmental)
    To visualize the coronary arterial system
    To determine the presence and severity of valvular stenosis/regurgitation
    To evaluate intracardiac shunts
    To evaluate congenital heart disease

Right Heart Catheterization

A catheter is inserted in an antecubital or femoral vein and advanced to the superior vena cava (SVC), inferior vena cava (IVC) right atrium (RA), right ventricle (RV), main pulmonary artery (MPA), and pulmonary artery wedge.

The following pressures are measured during a right heart catheterization:
    right atrial
    right ventricular systolic
    right ventricular end-diastolic
    systolic pulmonary artery
    pulmonary artery end-diastolic
    mean pulmonary artery
    pulmonary artery wedge

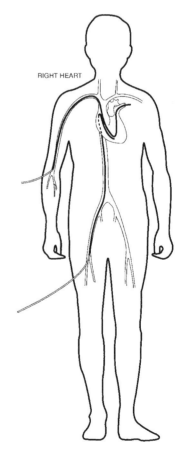

RIGHT HEART

During a right heart catheterization, oxygen saturations are determined by drawing blood samples from the SVC, IVC, RA, RV and MPA.

Left Heart Catheterization:

A left heart catheterization is performed by passing a catheter retrograde through the aorta into the left ventricle. This also permits measurement of pressures on either side of the aortic valve. The pressures measured are:

> Left ventricular systolic
> Left ventricular end-diastolic
> Aortic systolic/diastolic/mean

An aortogram may be performed during a left heart cardiac catheterization. A radiopaque dye is injected into the ascending aorta just above the aortic valve. If there is an incompetent aortic valve, a regurgitant jet of this radiopaque contrast material will be visible on the angiogram. The regurgitant jet is graded for severity from 1+ to 4+ with 1+ being mild regurgitation and 4+ being severe.

A left ventriculogram may be performed during a left heart catheterization. A contrast material is injected into the left ventricle. This permits visualization of global and segmental left ventricular function. Additionally, the severity of mitral regurgitation may be assessed by visualizing how much contrast material enters the left atrium. The mitral regurgitation is then graded 1+ to 4+ with 1+ being mild regurgitation and 4+ being severe.

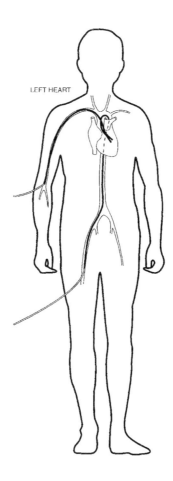

LEFT HEART

CHAPTER 5 (UNIT FIVE) - CARDIAC EVALUATION METHODS

REVIEW PRACTICE - Section 5E

1. _____ _____ is an invasive procedure used to visualize cardiac chambers and the coronary arterial system by introducing a catheter into the heart and great vessels.

2. Check the following if a possible objective of a cardiac catheterization:
    _____obtain intracardiac pressures/02 saturations
    _____assess ventricular function
    _____visualize the coronary arterial system
    _____determine the presence and severity of valvular regurgitation/stenosis
    _____evaluate intracardiac shunts
    _____evaluate congenital heart disease

3. True or False: A cardiac catheterization is performed by inserting a catheter into the right and left heart chambers where pressure measurements and blood samples are recorded.

4. Check the following if a possible place where a catheter is passed during a right heart catheterization:
    _____antecubital/femoral vein
    _____superior vena cava
    _____inferior vena cava
    _____right atrium
    _____right ventricle
    _____main pulmonary artery
    _____pulmonary artery wedge

5. Check the following if a possible pressure evaluated during a right heart catheterization:
    _____right atrium
    _____right ventricular systolic
    _____right ventricular end-diastolic
    _____systolic pulmonary artery
    _____pulmonary artery end-diastolic
    _____mean pulmonary artery
    _____pulmonary artery wedge

6. True or False: During a right heart catheterization blood samples are taken from the superior vena cava, inferior vena cava, right atrium, right ventricle and main pulmonary artery to determine oxygen saturations.

7. During a right heart catheterization, cardiac output may be determined by the _____ technique.

8. A _____ heart catheterization is performed by passing a catheter retrograde through the aorta into the left ventricle.

9. Check the following if a possible pressure measurement during a left heart catheterization:

    _____left ventricular systolic

    _____left ventricular end-diastolic

    _____aortic systolic

    _____aortic diastolic

    _____aortic mean

10. During a left heart catheterization, an _____ may be performed by injecting a radiopaque dye into the ascending aorta just above the aortic valve.

11. During left heart catheterization, a left _____ examination may be performed by injecting a radiopaque dye into the left ventricle.

12. A coronary _____ examines the coronary arteries by injecting a radiopaque dye into the ostia of each coronary artery.

13. True or False: A reduction of the diameter of a coronary artery diameter by 70% or more is considered significant coronary artery disease.

BOARD REVIEW QUESTIONS - Section 5E

1. Which of the following examinations is an invasive procedure used to visualize cardiac chambers and the coronary arterial system?
    a. echocardiography
    b. electrocardiography
    c. electroencephalogram
    d. cardiac catheterization

2. All of the following may be assessed during a cardiac catheterization except:
    a. intracardiac pressures
    b. oxygen saturations
    c. ventricular function
    d. pericardial thickness

3. All of the following may be assessed during a cardiac catheterization except:
    a. coronary arterial system
    b. valvular regurgitation/stenosis
    c. intracardiac shunts
    d. pulmonary function

4. All of the following may be catheterized during a right heart catheterization except:
    a. vena cava
    b. pulmonary veins
    c. right atrium
    d. pulmonary artery

5. All of the following pressures may be measured during a right heart catheterization except:
    a. right atrium
    b. right ventricle
    c. main pulmonary artery
    d. mean aortic

6. During a right heart catheterization, oxygen saturations may be obtained in each of the following except:
    a. vena cava
    b. pulmonary veins
    c. right atrium
    d. right ventricle

7. The most common method of determining cardiac output during a right heart cardiac catheterization procedure is the:
    a. Fick
    b. thermodilution
    c. indicator dye
    d. angiography

8. The cardiac catheterization procedure that allows calculation of pressures on either side of the aortic valve is the:
    a. right heart catheterization
    b. left heart catheterization
    c. pulmonary artery wedge
    d. coronary arteriogram

9. All of the following pressures may be measured during a left heart catheterization except:
    a. left ventricular systolic/diastolic
    b. aortic systolic/diastolic
    c. aortic mean
    d. pulmonary artery wedge

10. The left heart cardiac procedure that allows the evaluation of aortic regurgitation is:
    a. ventriculogram
    b. arteriogram
    c. aortogram
    d. venogram

11. The left heart cardiac catheterization procedure that allows for the evaluation of mitral regurgitation is:
    a. aortogram
    b. arteriogram
    c. venogram
    d. ventriculogram

12. The cardiac catheterization procedure that allows for the evaluation of the coronary arterial system is:
    a. aortogram
    b. arteriogram
    c. venogram
    d. ventriculogram

13. Significant coronary artery disease is considered present when the coronary artery diameter is reduced by at least:
    a. 30%
    b. 50%
    c. 70%
    d. 90%

CHAPTER 5 (UNIT FIVE) - CARDIAC EVALUATION METHODS

ANSWERS - Section 5E

Review practice answers

1. cardiac catheterization
2. all
3. True
4. all
5. all
6. True
7. thermodilution
8. left
9. all
10. aortogram
11. ventriculogram
12. arteriogram
13. True

Board review answers

1. d
2. d
3. d
4. b
5. d
6. b
7. b
8. b
9. d
10. c
11. d
12. b
13. c

Coronary Arteriography

Coronary artery catheterization is accomplished by inserting a special tipped catheter into the brachial artery (Sones approach) or femoral artery (Judkins approach) and advanced to the aortic root. The coronary catheter is introduced into the coronary orifice and contrast material injected. Coronary artery stenosis is graded from mild to severe. A 70% or greater reduction in a coronary artery diameter is considered significant.

A catheter is placed in the coronary ostia and radiopaque dye is injected with cine films recording the movement of the dye through the coronary arterial system. An abnormal coronary arteriogram is considered present when there is a greater than 70% diameter stenosis.

The left anterior descending artery provides blood flow to the anterior interventricular septum, anterior left ventricular wall and cardiac apex.

The left circumflex coronary artery provides blood flow to the left ventricular anterolateral and lateral walls. In a left dominant system, the left circumflex coronary will provide the posterior descending coronary artery which will provide blood to the inferior walls of the left and right ventricles and the inferior interventricular septum.

The right coronary artery provides blood flow to the right ventricle, sinoatrial node and atrioventricular node. In 67% of humans the right coronary artery is dominant, meaning that it provides the posterior descending coronary artery. The posterior descending coronary artery provides blood flow to the inferior walls of both ventricles and the inferior interventricular septum.

REVIEW PRACTICE - Section 5E

1. In coronary _____, a catheter is placed in the coronary artery ostia and a radiopaque dye is injected with cine films recording the movement of the dye through the coronary system.

2. A _____% or greater stenosis is considered significant coronary artery disease.

3. The left _____ descending coronary artery provides blood flow to the anterior interventricular septum and anterior wall of the left ventricle.

4. The left _____ coronary artery provides blood flow to the anterolateral and lateral walls of the left ventricle in a right dominant system.

5. In a left dominant coronary artery system the left anterior descending?/left circumflex?/right coronary artery? provides the posterior descending coronary artery.

6. The _____ coronary artery provides blood flow to the right ventricle.

7. In a right dominant coronary artery system, the _____descending coronary artery is a branch of the right coronary artery.

BOARD REVIEW QUESTIONS - Section 5E

1. Which of the following cardiac catheterization procedures is used to determine the percent stenosis of a coronary artery?
   a. arteriogram
   b. aortogram
   c. ventriculogram
   d. oximetry

2. Which percent stenosis is considered significant coronary artery disease?
   a. 10%
   b. 30%
   c. 50%
   d. 70%

3. Which of the following coronary arteries provides blood flow to the anterior interventricular septum and the anterior wall of the left ventricle?
   a. left main
   b. left anterior descending
   c. left circumflex
   d. posterior descending

4. Which of the following coronary arteries provides blood flow to the anterolateral and lateral walls of the left ventricle?
   a. left main
   b. left anterior descending
   c. left circumflex
   d. posterior descending

5. Which of the following coronary arteries provides blood flow to the right ventricle?
   a. left main
   b. anterior descending
   c. circumflex
   d. right coronary

6. Which of the following coronary arteries provides blood flow to the inferior walls of the ventricles and the inferior interventricular septum in a right dominant system?
   a. left main
   b. anterior descending
   c. circumflex
   d. posterior descending

7. In a left dominant coronary artery system, which of the following coronary arteries provides the posterior descending coronary artery?
   a. left main
   b. left anterior descending
   c. left circumflex
   d. right coronary artery

ANSWERS - Section 5E

Review practice answers

1. arteriography
2. 70
3. anterior
4. circumflex
5. left circumflex
6. right
7. posterior

Board review answers

1. a
2. d
3. b
4. c
5. d
6. d
7. c

Valve Area

DETERMINATION of VALVE AREAS:

The Gorlin equation is used to determine valve area during cardiac catheterization.

Mitral valve area(cm²) = CO/Diastolic filling period/38 x $\sqrt{MPG}$

Aortic valve area(cm²) = CO/Systolic ejection period/44.5 x $\sqrt{MPG}$

REVIEW PRACTICE - Section 5E

1.   The _____ formula is used to determine valve area in the cardiac catheterization laboratory.

2.   The Gorlin formula for mitral valve area is:

    MVA(cm²) = CO/diastolic flow/_____   x $\sqrt{MPG}$

3.   The Gorlin formula for aortic valve area is:

    AVA(cm²) = CO/systolic ejection period/_____   x $\sqrt{MPG}$

BOARD REVIEW QUESTIONS - Section 5E

1. The formula used to determine valve area in the cardiac catheterization laboratory is:
   a. Doppler
   b. Gorlin
   c. Bernoulli
   d. continuity

2. The formula used to determine mitral valve area in the cardiac catheterization laboratory is
   MVA (cm^2) =
   a. CSA x TVI
   b. $4 \times (V_2)^2$
   c. CO/DFP/38 x $\sqrt{MPG}$
   d. SV x HR

3. The formula used to determine the aortic valve area in the cardiac catheterization laboratory is:
   a. CSA x TVI
   b. $4 \times (V_2)^2$
   c. CO/SFP/44.5 x $\sqrt{MPG}$
   d. CO/DFP/38 x $\sqrt{MPG}$

ANSWERS - Section 5E

Review practice answers

1. Gorlin
2. 38
3. 44.5

Board review answers

1. b
2. c
3. c

2. DETERMINATION OF CARDIAC OUTPUT

The following methods may be used during a cardiac catheterization to determine cardiac output:

Thermodilution

Cardiac output is determined during a right heart catheterization using the thermodilution tecnique. This is the most common technique used currently. A chilled ($0°$ C) saline is injected into the right atrium and the temperature change is measured at the pulmonary artery. The temperature change is plotted on a graph over time which allows for the calculation of cardiac output.

Indicator Dilution

Indocyanine green dye is injected into the right heart and the concentration of dye is measured at a distal arterial site. The change in the concentration of dye is plotted on a graph over time and cardiac output is then derived from this plotted curve.

Fick Method

Considered the most accurate method for determining cardiac output, the Fick method compares oxygen consumption between the pulmonary system and the systemic system.

REVIEW PRACTICE - Section 5E

1. The most common invasive method used to determine cardiac output is the _____ technique.

2. The _____ method for predicting cardiac output uses the injection of chilled saline into the right atrium and detects the temperature change at the pulmonary artery.

3. The _____ _____ method is an invasive procedure used to determine cardiac output by injecting dye into the right heart and measuring the concentration of dye at a distal arterial site.

4. The most accurate invasive method of determining cardiac output is the _____ method.

5. An invasive procedure called _____ allows calculation of cardiac output by injecting a radiopaque dye into the left ventricle.

BOARD REVIEW QUESTIONS - Section 5E

1. The most common invasive method of determining cardiac output is:
   a. Fick
   b. thermodilution
   c. indicator dilution
   d. angiography

2. Which invasive method to determine cardiac output measures the concentration of dye that has been injected into the right heart and measured at a distal arterial site?
   a. Fick
   b. thermodilution
   c. indicator dilution
   d. angiography

3. Which of the following invasive methods used to determine cardiac output is considered to be the most accurate?
   a. Fick
   b. thermodilution
   c. indicator dilution
   d. angiography

4. Which of the following invasive techniques determine cardiac output by injecting dye into the left ventricle and measuring ventricular volumes?
   a. Fick
   b. thermodilution
   c. indicator dilution
   d. angiography

ANSWERS - Section 5E

Review practice answers

1. thermodilution
2. thermodilution
3. indicator dilution
4. Fick
5. angiography

Board review answers

1. b
2. c
3. a
4. d

3. OXIMETRY

During a cardiac catheterization, measurement of the oxygen content in the right heart is performed. A 10% difference in oxygen saturation from one chamber to the next may indicate the presence of a left to right shunt.

For example, the following oxygen saturations were determined during a right heart catheterization:
Vena cava: 72%
Right atrium: 72%
Right ventricle: 85%
Main pulmonary artery: 85%

There is a 13% oxygen step-up in the right ventricle, suggesting the presence of a left-to-right ventricular septal defect shunt.

Selective angiography is another method used to evaluate left to right shunts by visualizing and localizing the site of the shunt.

During a cardiac catheterization, a regurgitant volume and regurgitant fraction may be determined. The formula is:

Regurgitant volume = total stroke volume - forward stroke volume

where total stroke volume is the blood flow volume across the regurgitant valve and the forward stroke volume is the blood flow across a non-regurgitant valve.

A regurgitant fraction may be derived by the formula:

Regurgitant fraction = regurgitant volume/total stroke volume

REVIEW PRACTICE - Section 5E

1. True or False: An oxygen step-up of 10% or greater may indicate the presence of a left-to-right shunt.

2. Examine the oxygen saturations obtained during a cardiac catheterization shown below. Is there a left-to-right shunt present?

   Yes?/No?
   > Superior vena cava: 72%
   > Inferior vena cava: 78%
   > Right atrium: 86%
   > Right ventricle: 86%
   > Main pulmonary artery: 86%

3. The diagnosis for the above case is_____ _____ defect.

4. Examine the oxygen saturations obtained during a cardiac catheterization shown below. Is there a left-to-right shunt present?

   Yes?/No?
   > Superior vena cava: 72%
   > Inferior vena cava: 78%
   > Right atrium: 75%
   > Right ventricle: 86%
   > Main pulmonary artery: 86%

5. The diagnosis for question #4 is:_____ _____ defect.

6. Examine the oxygen saturations obtained during a cardiac catheterization shown below. Is there a left-to-right shunt present?

   Yes?/No?
   > Superior vena cava: 72%
   > Inferior vena cava: 78%
   > Right atrium: 75%
   > Right ventricle: 75%
   > Main pulmonary artery: 88%

7. The diagnosis for #6 question is: _____ _____   _____.

8. The formula that may be used to determine regurgitant volume during a cardiac catheterization is: regurgitant volume (cc) _____ stroke volume -_____ stroke volume.

9. The flow through the mitral valve is determined to be 100 cc. The flow through the aortic valve is determined to be 50 cc. The mitral regurgitant volume is:_____cc.

10. The formula used to determine regurgitant fraction during a cardiac catheterization is: regurgitant fraction% = _____ stroke volume / _____ stroke volume.

11. For question #9, the mitral regurgitant fraction is:_____%.

BOARD REVIEW QUESTIONS - Section 5E

1. Which of the following procedures during a cardiac catheterization allows for the detection of an intracardiac shunt?
   a. aortography
   b. arteriography
   c. oximetry
   d. pressure waveforms

2. The following oxygen saturations have been recorded:
   Superior vena cava: 72%
   Inferior vena cava: 78%
   Right atrium: 87%
   Right ventricle: 87%
   Main pulmonary artery: 87%

   The diagnosis is:
   a. normal
   b. atrial septal defect
   c. ventricular septal defect
   d. patent ductus arteriosus

3. The following oxygen saturations have been recorded:
   Superior vena cava: 72%
   Inferior vena cava: 78%
   Right atrium: 75%
   Right ventricle: 85%
   Main pulmonary artery: 85%

   The diagnosis is:
   a. normal
   b. atrial septal defect
   c. ventricular defect
   d. patent ductus arteriosus

4. The following oxygen saturations have been recorded:
    Superior vena cava: 72%
    Inferior vena cava: 78%
    Right atrium: 75%
    Right ventricle: 75%
    Main pulmonary artery: 89%

    The diagnosis is:
    a. normal
    b. atrial septal defect
    c. ventricular septal defect
    d. patent ductus arteriosus

5. The forward flow across a normal valve is determined to be 60 cc. The total stroke volume across a regurgitant valve is 120 cc. The regurgitant volume is:
    a. 0 cc
    b. 60 cc
    c. 120 cc
    d. 180 cc

6. The regurgitant fraction for question number 5 is:
    a. 0%
    b. 50%
    c. 60%
    d. 90%

ANSWERS - Section 5E

Review practice answers

1. True
2. Yes
3. atrial septal
4. Yes
5. ventricular septal
6. Yes
7. patent ductus arteriosus
8. total, forward
9. 50 cc
10. regurgitant, total
11. 50

Board review answers

1. c
2. b
3. c
4. d
5. b
6. b

4. ANGIOGRAPHY

Angiography is the injection of radiopaque dye into cardiac chambers and great vessels and recording the movement of the dye through the cardiac chambers and vessels on cine film.

Left Ventricular Angiography

Also called left ventriculography, it is the injection of a radiopaque dye into the left ventricle as part of a left heart catheterization. The following may be evaluated:

Left ventricular function (e.g., ejection fraction, stroke volume, cardiac output)

Regional wall motion abnormalities

The severity of mitral regurgitation may be evaluated by injecting radiopaque dye into the left ventricle and grading the amount that regurgitates into the left atrium. The severity range is from grade 1+ (mild) to grade 4+ (severe).

Right Ventricular Angiography

Also may be referred to as right ventriculography, a catheter is placed into the right ventricle and an injection of a radiopaque dye is performed. A right ventriculogram allows for the evaluation of:

Right ventricular global and segmental systolic function.

Tricuspid regurgitation

Aortography

An injection of radiopaque dye into the ascending aorta is performed and the amount that regurgitates across the aortic valve is evaluated. The severity is graded from mild (1+) to severe (4+).

Pulmonary Artery Arteriography

A radiopaque dye is injected into the pulmonary artery to rule out pulmonary thrombosis or pulmonary artery stenosis.

REVIEW PRACTICE - Section 5E

1. _____ is the injection of radiopaque dye into cardiac chambers/great vessels and recorded on cine film.

2. Ventricular _____ or ventriculography is the injection of a radiopaque dye into the ventricle during a left heart catheterization.

3. Check the following if a left ventricular angiogram (ventriculogram) would be used for evaluation of the items listed below:

    _____ ejection fraction
    _____ stroke volume
    _____ cardiac output
    _____ cardiac index
    _____ regional wall motion abnormalities
    _____ mitral regurgitation

4. True or False: Right ventricular angiography (ventriculography) is the injection of a radiopaque dye into the right ventricle during a right heart catheterization.

5. Check the following if a right ventricular angiogram (ventriculogram) allows for evaluation for:

    _____right ventricular function
    _____tricuspid regurgitation

6. _____ is the injection of a radiopaque dye into the ascending aorta in order to evaluate aortic regurgitation.

7. True or False: A pulmonary artery arteriogram is the injection of a radiopaque dye into the main pulmonary artery in order to rule out pulmonary thrombosis or pulmonary artery stenosis.

BOARD REVIEW QUESTIONS - Section 5E

1. The cardiac catheterization examination that injects a radiopaque dye into cardiac chambers/great vessels and is recorded on cine film is (a):
   a. angiography
   b. contrast study
   c. hemodynamic recording
   d. ejection fraction

2. Which of the following cardiac catheterization exams allows for the evaluation of ventricular function parameters (i.e..ejection fraction, stroke volume, cardiac output, cardiac index), regional wall motion abnormalities and atrioventricular regurgitation?
   a. arteriography
   b. angiography
   c. radiography
   d. Doppler

3. Which of the following cardiac catheterization exams allows for the evaluation of aortic regurgitation?
   a. angiography
   b. arteriography
   c. aortography
   d. ventriculogram

4. Which of the following cardiac catheterization exams allows for the evaluation of pulmonary artery stenosis and pulmonary thrombosis?
   a. cardiac Doppler
   b. aortography
   c. ventriculography
   d. angiography

ANSWERS - Section 5E

Review practice answers

1. angiography
2. angiography
3. all
4. True
5. all
6. aortography
7. True

Board review answers

1. a
2. b
3. c
4. d

5. EVALUATION AND DEFINITION OF GRADIENTS

A pressure gradient is the pressure difference between two chambers. The cardiac catheterization laboratory measures gradients three ways:

Peak to Peak: The peak to peak method compares the peak systolic pressure of the right ventricle or left ventricle to the peak systolic pressure of the pulmonary artery or aorta respectively. This is used to determine the severity of semilunar valve stenosis. Cardiac Doppler does not allow for the calculation of the peak to peak gradient.

Mean: The mean gradient measures the pressure gradient over time. The mean gradient is used to assess valvular stenosis. Cardiac Doppler and the cardiac catheterization's mean gradient should demonstrate close correlation.

Peak instantaneous: The peak instantaneous pressure gradient is measured at the peak pressure difference between two cardiac chambers. This value may be expressed when evaluating valvular stenosis. Cardiac Doppler may also be used to predict the peak instantaneous pressure gradient.

IMPORTANT TO NOTE

When comparing cardiac catheterization gradients with cardiac Doppler gradients, it is important to remember that there will be a close correlation in the mean gradients. There will be a poor correlation when comparing the peak to peak gradient to either the cardiac Doppler mean or peak instantaneous gradient.

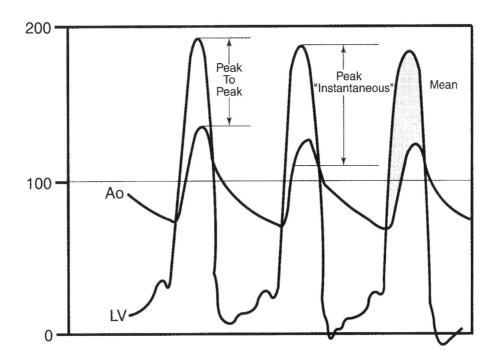

CHAPTER 5 (UNIT FIVE) - CARDIAC EVALUATION METHODS

2. The cardiac catheterization laboratory measures pressure gradients three ways. They are: 1._____ to _____, 2._____ , and 3. _____ instantaneous.

3. The _____ to _____ method compares the peak systolic pressure of the left or right ventricle to the peak systolic pressure of the respective great artery.

4. The _____ pressure gradient represents the average pressure gradient.

5. The _____ _____ pressure gradient represents the maximum pressure gradient between two cardiac chambers.

6. The _____ gradient of a cardiac Doppler examination will correlate best with the cardiac catheterization mean gradient.

7. True or False: The peak to peak cardiac catheterization gradient will correlate closely with the cardiac Doppler peak instantaneous gradient.

8. A cardiac Doppler examination demonstrates a peak instantaneous pressure gradient across the aortic valve of 66 mm Hg. The cardiac catheterization peak to peak gradient will be higher?/equal to/lower? than the cardiac Doppler gradient?

CHAPTER 5 (UNIT FIVE) - CARDIAC EVALUATION METHODS

BOARD REVIEW QUESTIONS- Section 5E

1. The difference in pressures between two cardiac chambers is called a pressure:
   a. velocity
   b. gradient
   c. area
   d. increase

2. The cardiac catheterization laboratory may express a pressure gradient all of the following ways except:
   a. peak to peak
   b. peak to mean
   c. peak instantaneous
   d. mean

3. The pressure gradient measurement that expresses the difference between the peak systolic pressure of a ventricle and a great artery is the:
   a. peak
   b. peak to peak
   c. peak instantaneous
   d. mean

4. The pressure gradient that expresses the average pressure gradient between two chambers is the:
   a. peak
   b. peak to peak
   c. peak instantaneous
   d. mean

5. The pressure gradient that expresses the maximum gradient between two chambers is:
   a. mean
   b. peak to mean
   c. peak to peak
   d. peak instantaneous

6. Which of the following cardiac Doppler measurements would correlate best with the cardiac catheterization gradient measurement?
   a. peak velocity
   b. peak instantaneous
   c. mean
   d. peak to peak

7. A patient with valvular aortic stenosis has a peak instantaneous gradient of 100 mm Hg. The cardiac catheterization peak to peak gradient is 60 mm Hg. The reason for the difference in the gradients is:

    a. cardiac Doppler is unreliable

    b. cardiac catheterization is a tarnished gold standard

    c. the Doppler peak instantaneous gradient will always be greater than the catheterization peak to peak

    d. the difference cannot be explained

ANSWERS - Section 5E

Review practice answers

1. gradient
2. peak to peak, mean, peak
3. peak, peak
4. mean
5. peak instantaneous
6. mean
7. False
8. lower

Board review answers

1. b
2. b
3. b
4. d
5. d
6. c
7. c

6. RECOGNITION OF PRESSURE WAVEFORMS IN COMMON DISEASE STATES

Mitral/tricuspid stenosis: In atrioventricular stenosis, the atrial pressure increases causing a pressure gradient to persist throughout ventricular diastole. (shaded area)

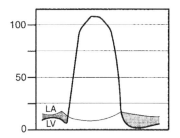 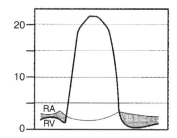

Mitral/tricuspid regurgitation: In atrioventricular regurgitation, the atrial pressure tracing will reflect an increase during ventricular systole of the atrial v wave.

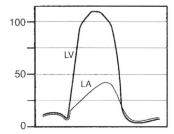 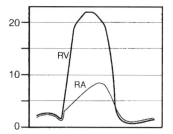

Aortic/Pulmonic valve stenosis: In semilunar valve stenosis, the ventricular systolic pressure increases creating a systolic pressure gradient between the ventricle and great artery. (see shaded area in diagram below)

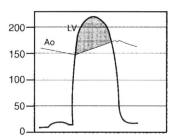 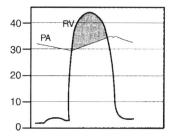

Aortic/Pulmonic regurgitation: In semilunar valve regurgitation, the arterial diastolic pressure decreases throughout diastole, thus decreasing the diastolic pressure gradient between the artery and ventricle.

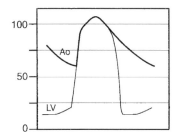 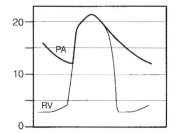

REVIEW PRACTICE - Section 5E

1.   Examine the pressure waveforms below. The diagnosis is:_____.

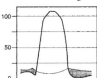

2.   Examine the pressure waveforms below. The diagnosis is:_____.

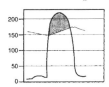

3.   Examine the pressure waveforms below. The diagnosis is:_____.

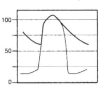

4.   Examine the pressure waveforms below. The diagnosis is:_____.

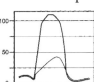

5.   Examine the pressure gradients below. The diagnosis is:_____.

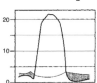

6.   Examine the pressure waveforms below. The diagnosis is:_____.

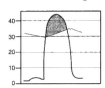

7.   Examine the pressure waveforms below. The diagnosis is:_____.

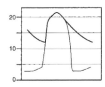

8.   Examine the pressure waveforms below. The diagnosis is:_____.

CHAPTER 5 (UNIT FIVE) - CARDIAC EVALUATION METHODS

BOARD REVIEW QUESTIONS - Section 5E

1. The pressure waveforms below demonstrate:
    a. mitral stenosis
    b. tricuspid stenosis
    c. mitral regurgitation
    d. tricuspid regurgitation

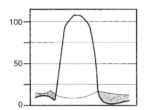

2. The pressure waveforms below is demonstrating:
    a. mitral stenosis
    b. tricuspid stenosis
    c. mitral regurgitation
    d. tricuspid regurgitation

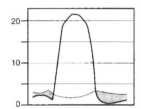

3. The pressure waveforms below are demonstrating:
    a. mitral regurgitation
    b. tricuspid regurgitation
    c. tricuspid stenosis
    d. mitral stenosis

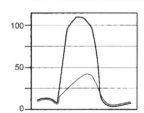

4. The pressure waveforms below are demonstrating:
    a. mitral regurgitation
    b. tricuspid regurgitation
    c. tricuspid stenosis
    d. pulmonic stenosis

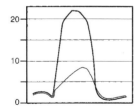

5.   The pressure waveforms below are demonstrating:
    a.   aortic stenosis
    b.   pulmonic stenosis
    c.   mitral regurgitation
    d.   aortic regurgitation

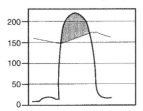

6.   The pressure waveforms below are demonstrating:
    a.   aortic stenosis
    b.   pulmonic stenosis
    c.   tricuspid regurgitation
    d.   pulmonic regurgitation

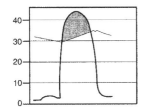

7.   The pressure waveforms below are demonstrating:
    a.   aortic stenosis
    b.   aortic regurgitation
    c.   mitral regurgitation
    d.   pulmonic regurgitation

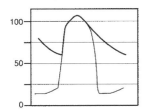

8.   The pressure waveforms below are demonstrating:
    a.   pulmonic stenosis
    b.   pulmonic regurgitation
    c.   aortic regurgitation
    d.   tricuspid regurgitation

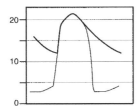

CHAPTER 5 (UNIT FIVE) - CARDIAC EVALUATION METHODS

ANSWERS - Section 5E

Review practice answers

1. mitral stenosis
2. vavular aortic stenosis
3. aortic regurgitation
4. mitral regurgitation
5. tricuspid stenosis
6. valvular pulmonic stenosis
7. pulmonic regurgitation
8. tricuspid regurgitation

Board review answers

1. a
2. b
3. a
4. b
5. a
6. b
7. b
8. b

SECTION 5F
Other Diagnostic Modalities

1. CHEST X-RAY

There are two common projections used to evaluate the heart. They are: posterior-anterior (PA) and left lateral. The chest x-ray findings that are helpful in detecting heart disease includes:

Cardiomegaly: An increase in heart size on the chest x-ray may suggest the presence of pericardial effusion, dilated cardiomyopathy, chamber hypertrophy and/or chamber dilatation. These findings can be confirmed during an echocardiographic examination.

Increased pulmonary vascularity: There are three types of increased pulmonary vascularity on chest x-ray. The first type is due to primary or secondary pulmonary artery hypertension. The classic pulmonary artery hypertension pattern is central arterial enlargement with abrupt peripheral arterial constriction. The second type of increased pulmonary vascularity is shunt vascularity due to atrial septal defect, ventricular septal defect or patent ductus arteriosus. With shunt vascularity an even increase in all vessels is seen in both lungs and the lungs are said to be overperfused.

The third type of increased pulmonary vascularity is called pulmonary venous hypertension which is the result of increased left atrial pressure such as in mitral valve stenosis or left ventricular failure. Pulmonary venous hypertension is demonstrated on the upright chest x-ray as vascular redistribution into the upper lobes termed cephalization of flow.

Cardiac Pathologies

Coronary Artery Disease: There are no specific chest x-ray findings for coronary artery disease. Left ventricular enlargement may be seen and may indicate decreased left ventricular systolic function. A left ventricular bulge suggests a left ventricular aneurysm.

Mitral Stenosis: On chest x-ray, the left atrium will be enlarged in a patient with mitral valve stenosis. Long standing mitral valve stenosis will lead to pulmonary venous hypertension, pulmonary arterial hypertension and right ventricular enlargement due to dilatation.

Mitral Regurgitation: Significant chronic mitral regurgitation will cause the left atrium and left ventricle to appear enlarged on chest x-ray due to chamber dilatation.

Aortic Regurgitation: On a chest x-ray, significant chronic aortic regurgitation will cause the left ventricle to appear enlarged and elongated due to ventricular dilatation.

Valvular Aortic Stenosis: Concentric left ventricular hypertrophy will cause the left ventricle to appear enlarged with blunting of the cardiac apex. Post-stenotic dilatation of the aorta is also associated with valvular aortic stenosis.

Atrial Septal Defect: Atrial septal defect will cause an increase in pulmonary vascularity, main pulmonary artery dilatation, right atrial and right ventricular enlargement due to chamber dilatation.

Ventricular Septal Defect: On chest x-ray a ventricular septal defect will cause an increase in pulmonary vascularity. The main pulmonary artery will be prominent and the left atrium and left ventricle will appear enlarged due to chamber dilatation.

Patent Ductus Arteriosus: On chest x-ray, patent ductus arteriosus will cause an increase in pulmonary vascularity. The left atrium and left ventricle will appear enlarged due to chamber dilatation.

Valvular Pulmonic Valve Stenosis: On chest x-ray, valvular pulmonic stenosis is associated with right ventricular enlargement due to right ventricular hypertrophy. Valvular pulmonic stenosis may cause post stenotic dilatation of the pulmonary artery.

Coarctation of the Aorta: Coarctation is associated with cardiac enlargement due to left ventricular hypertrophy, the figure three sign and rib notching.

Pericardial Effusion: By chest x- ray pericardial effusion creates an increase in the cardiac silhouette. At least 200 cc of pericardial fluid is necessary before cardiac enlargement is apparent.

Miscellaneous Chest X-Ray Findings

The following findings may be seen on a chest x-ray examination: aortic dilatation, pleural effusion, a widened mediastinum (associated with aortic dissection or tumor), calcified pericardium (associated with constrictive pericarditis) and pacemaker placement. These findings may be confirmed during a routine echocardiographic examination. Transesophageal echocardiography is helpful in cases where aortic dissection or mediastinal tumor may be present.

REVIEW PRACTICE - Section 5F

1. Two common chest x-ray projections that may be helpful for evaluating the heart are the
    _____-_____ and the _____ _____.

2. True or False: Cardiomegaly by chest x-ray may indicate the presence of pericardial effusion, dilated cardiomyopathy and/or ventricular hypertrophy/dilatation.

3. True or False: The three types of increased pulmonary vascularity seen on chest x-ray are pulmonary arterial hypertension, shunt vascularity and pulmonary venous hypertension.

4. True or False: The classic pulmonary artery hypertension pattern seen on chest x-ray is central arterial enlargement with abrupt peripheral arterial constriction.

5. The second type of increased pulmonary vascularity as seen on chest x-ray is called _____ vascularity due to an atrial septal defect, ventricular septal defect or patent ductus arteriosus.

6. The third type of increased pulmonary vascularity as seen on chest x-ray is called pulmonary _____ hypertension due to an increase in left atrial pressure.

7. True or False: There are no specific chest x-ray findings for coronary artery disease, although left ventricular enlargement may be seen and suggests decreased left ventricular systolic function.

8. A left ventricular bulge seen on a chest x-ray may indicate the presence of a left ventricular _____.

9. A possible chest x-ray finding for mitral valve stenosis is left atrial _____ due to chamber enlargement..

10. On chest x-ray significant, chronic mitral valve regurgitation may cause left _____ and left atrial enlargement due to chamber dilatation.

11. True or False: Significant chronic aortic regurgitation will cause the left ventricle to appear enlarged and elongated due to ventricular dilatation on chest x-ray.

12. True or False: Valvular aortic stenosis leads to concentric left ventricular hypertrophy, causing the left ventricle to appear enlarged and the cardiac apex to be blunted on chest x-ray.

13. _____ stenotic dilatation of the ascending aorta may be seen on a chest x-ray of a patient with valvular aortic stenosis.

14. The chest x-ray findings for atrial septal defect includes an increase?/decrease? in pulmonary vascularity, main pulmonary artery dilatation and right ventricular enlargement.

15. A patent ductus arteriosus may cause dilatation of the main pulmonary artery, left _____ and left ventricle.

16. On chest x-ray, valvular pulmonic stenosis may cause right ventricular enlargement due to right ventricular hypertrophy and post stenotic dilatation of the main pulmonary artery.

17. True or False: The chest x-ray findings for aortic coarctation include left ventricular enlargement due to left ventricular hypertrophy, the figure three sign and/or rib notching.

18. Pericardial effusion causes an increase?/decrease? of the cardiac silhouette on chest x-ray.

19. Check the following if possible to assess by chest x-ray:

_____aortic dilatation

_____pleural effusion

_____widened mediastinum

_____aortic dissection

_____tumor

_____calcified pericardium

20. Check the following if possible to assess by echocardiography/Doppler:

_____pericardial effusion

_____dilated cardiomyopathy

_____ventricular hypertrophy/dilatation

_____left heart failure

_____left to right shunt

_____valvular heart disease

_____aortic dilatation

_____pleural effusion

_____aortic dissection

_____constrictive pericarditis

BOARD REVIEW QUESTIONS - Section 5F

1. Which of the following chest x-ray projections is useful in evaluating the heart?
    a. posterior-anterior
    b. lateral
    c. anterior oblique
    d. right lateral

2. Cardiomegaly on chest x-ray is associated with all of the following except:
    a. pericardial effusion
    b. ventricular hypertrophy/dilatation
    c. acute myocardial infarction
    d. dilated cardiomyopathy

3. All of the following are types of increased pulmonary vascularity as seen on chest x-ray except:
    a. pulmonary artery hypertension
    b. shunt vascularity
    c. pulmonary venous hypertension
    d. pulmonary embolism

4. The chest x-ray findings for coronary artery disease is/are:
    a. left atrial enlargement
    b. right ventricular enlargement
    c. figure 3 sign
    d. nonspecific

5. A left ventricular bulge on chest x-ray may indicate the presence of a left ventricular:
    a. thrombus
    b. aneurysm
    c. infarction
    d. normal ventricle

6. All of the following chambers may appear enlarged on a chest x-ray of a patient with mitral valve stenosis except:
    a. left atrium
    b. left ventricle
    c. right ventricle
    d. right atrium

7. Which of the following cardiac chambers would most likely appear enlarged on chest x-ray in a patient with mitral regurgitation?
    a. left atrium, right atrium
    b. left ventricle, right ventricle
    c. left atrium, left ventricle
    d. right atrium, right ventricle

8. The most likely chest x-ray finding in a patient with significant chronic aortic regurgitation is enlargement of the:
    a. left atrium
    b. left ventricle
    c. right atrium
    d. right ventricle

9. The chest x-ray finding of left ventricular enlargement due to concentric left ventricular hypertrophy, blunting of the cardiac apex and post stenotic dilatation of the ascending aorta most likely indicates:
    a. mitral valve stenosis
    b. significant,chronic mitral regurgitation
    c. valvular aortic stenosis
    d. significant, chronic aortic regurgitation

10. All of the following are possible chest x ray findings for atrial septal defect except:
    a. right ventricular enlargement
    b. main pulmonary artery enlargement
    c. figure 3 sign
    d. increased pulmonary vascularity

11. All of the following are possible chest x ray findings for patent ductus arteriosus except:
    a. increased pulmonary vascularity
    b. left atrial enlargement
    c. left ventricular enlargement
    d. rib notching

12. Right ventricular enlargement due to right ventricular hypertrophy and post stenotic dilatation of the main pulmonary artery on chest x ray is most likely associated with:
    a. valvular aortic stenosis
    b. valvular pulmonic stenosis
    c. mitral valve stenosis
    d. mitral regurgitation

13. All of the following chest x-ray findings are associated with coarctation of the aorta except:
    a. left ventricular enlargement
    b. right ventricular enlargement
    c. figure three sign
    d. rib notching

CHAPTER 5 (UNIT FIVE) - CARDIAC EVALUATION METHODS

14. Which of the following is associated with an increase of the cardiac silhouette as seen on chest x-ray?
    a. pleural effusion
    b. constrictive pericarditis
    c. pericardial effusion
    d. aortic aneurysm

15. All of the following may be diagnosed by chest x-ray except:
    a. aortic dilatation/aortic dissection
    b. pleural effusion
    c. myocardial ischemia
    d. calcified pericardium

ANSWERS - Section 5F

Review practice answers

1. posterior, anterior, left lateral
2. True
3. True
4. True
5. shunt
6. venous
7. True
8. aneurysm
9. enlargement
10. ventricular
11. True
12. True
13. post
14. increase
15. atrium
16. True
17. True
18. increase
19. all
20. all

Board review answers

1. a
2. c
3. d
4. d
5. b
6. b
7. c
8. b
9. c
10. c
11. d
12. b
13. b
14. c
15. c

2. NUCLEAR CARDIOLOGY

Nuclear cardiology involves the injection of radioisotopes into the body. These isotopes are selectively absorbed by certain tissues of the body. The concentration of isotope is detected with a gamma recorder.

Types of Nuclear Cardiology Exams

Myocardial perfusion: Myocardial perfusion imaging assesses myocardial blood flow by using radioisotopes that are injected into the blood stream and accumulate in the myocardium. Thallium 201 is a common radioisotope used for myocardial perfusion. Thallium 201 is accumulated in areas of viable myocardium in proportion to blood flow to those regions. Areas where there is decreased blood flow are represented by decreased or absent thallium uptake and are seen as cold spots. The most common application of Thallium 201 myocardial perfusion imaging is during a stress test.

Approximately one minute before stopping the exercise portion of the stress test, Thallium 201 is injected intravenously and the patient is sent to the nuclear cardiology laboratory where the patient is scanned by a gamma scintillation camera. There will be diminished Thallium uptake in areas of decreased blood flow. Three to four hours later the patient is rescanned. If the cold spots that were seen immediate post exercise disappear, this indicates myocardial ischemia. If the cold spots persist myocardial scar or old infarction is present. A new isotope, Technetium-99m sestamibi (Cardiolyte) may also be used to detect coronary artery disease similar to Thallium.

Infarct avid imaging: The isotope 99m technetium pyrophosphate is a radioactive material used to diagnose acute myocardial infarction. The isotope is injected into the patient 12 hours to 6 days after symptoms arise and a scintillation camera scans the heart. Injured areas of the heart appear as bright areas (hot spots). The size of the spot corresponds to the size of the injury.

Radionuclide angiography: The isotope technetium 99m is injected which allows visualization of the atria, ventricles and great vessels. There are two types of radionuclide angiography: first pass and gated equilibrium. The first pass study records the radioactivity in the heart for a single beat. This is played back similar to a motion picture. The gated study records several hundred cardiac cycles until a recurrent pattern of images demonstrate cardiac wall motion.

The radionuclide angiography exam permits the accurate evaluation of ejection fraction and regional wall motion abnormalities during rest and exercise. Radionuclide angiography may also be referred to as multiple gated acquisition scanning (MUGA), blood pool imaging, gated heart study or wall motion study.

REVIEW PRACTICE - Section 5F

1. True or False: Nuclear cardiology involves the injection of radioisotopes to obtain cardiac images.

2. In the nuclear cardiology test called _____ _____, a radioisotope such as Thallium-201 is injected at peak exercise to evaluate for coronary artery disease.

3. In Thallium-201 testing infarcted or ischemic tissue is represented as a cold?/hot? spot.

4. In the nuclear cardiology test called _____ _____ imaging, the isotope technetium 99 pyrophosphate is injected in order to detect infarcted myocardial tissue.

5. In infarct avid imaging infarcted tissue appears as a cold?/hot? spot.

6. In the nuclear cardiology test _____ _____, the isotope technetium 99m is injected to visualize the atria, ventricles and great vessels.

7. True or False: The MUGA scan allows for accurate evaluation of ejection fraction.

BOARD REVIEW QUESTIONS - Section 5F

1. Which of the following nuclear cardiology isotopes would be best to use to rule out a decrease in myocardial perfusion?
   a. Thallium-201
   b. technetium-99
   c. pyrophosphate
   d. Albunex

2. Which of the following nuclear cardiology isotopes would be best to use to evaluate ejection fraction?
   a. Thallium 201
   b. technetium-99
   c. Cardiolyte
   d. Albunex

3. Which of the following nuclear cardiology isotopes would be best to use to image infarcted myocardium?
   a. Thallium-201
   b. Technetium-99
   c. Cardiolyte
   d. pyrophosphate

4. Which of the following noninvasive examinations is also called cold spot scanning?
   a. myocardial perfusion
   b. infarct avid imaging
   c. radionuclide angiography
   d. MUGA

5. Which of the following nuclear studies is also referred to as hot spot scanning?
   a. myocardial perfusion
   b. infarct avid imaging
   c. radionuclide angiography
   d. MUGA

ANSWERS - Section 5F

Review practice answers

1. True
2. myocardial perfusion
3. cold
4. infarct avid
5. hot
6. radionuclide angiography
7. True

Board review answers

1. a
2. b
3. d
4. a
5. b

CHAPTER SIX
PRINCIPLES OF CARDIAC HEMODYNAMICS

SECTION A.   Blood Flow Dynamics

SECTION B.   Effects of Abnormal Pressures and Loading

SECTION 6A
Blood Flow Dynamics

1. FACTORS AFFECTING BLOOD FLOW

The factors that govern the flow of fluids (including blood) include the pressure gradient, the radius of the tube the fluid is flowing in, the length of the tube and the viscosity of the fluid. These factors are expressed in Poiseuille's law.

Poiseuille's Law

Poiseuille's law states that flow volume (Q) varies directly with the pressure gradient (Pi-Po) and the fourth power of the radius of the tube (r). Flow (Q) varies inversely with the length (L) of the tube and the viscosity (n) of a fluid.

Poiseuille's law may be written: $Q = (Pi\text{-}Po)\pi r^4 /8nL$

Poiseuille's law can be interpreted as follows:
    As the pressure gradient increases, flow volume increases.
    As the tube diameter increases, flow volume increases.
    As the length of the tube increases, flow volume decreases.
    As fluid viscosity increases, flow volume decreases.

It is important to note that a tube's diameter (radius) is to the fourth power and thus exerts the greatest influence on flow volume.

Since the viscosity of blood and the length of blood vessels do not vary significantly in the cardiovascular system, it is the changes in the vessel radius and pressure gradient that are most significant.

Resistance

Poiseuille's formula may be rearranged to predict the resistance to flow through a tube:

$$R = 8nL/\pi r^4$$

where R is overall flow resistance, n is viscosity of the fluid, L is the length of the tube and r is the radius of the tube.

An increase in fluid viscosity and/or tube length will increase resistance. A change in the radius of a tube exerts the greatest influence on resistance.

REVIEW PRACTICE - Section 6A

1. True or False: The factors that affect flow volume (Q) include the pressure gradient, tube radius, tube length and fluid viscosity.

2. According to Poiseuille's law, flow volume varies directly?/indirectly? with pressure gradient.

3. According to Poiseuille's law, flow volume varies directly?/indirectly? with tube radius.

4. True or False: According to Poiseuille's law, flow volume varies inversely with tube length.

5. True or False: According to Poiseuille's law, flow volume varies inversely with fluid viscosity.

6. True or False: As the pressure gradient increases, flow volume increases.

7. True or False: As the pressure gradient decreases, flow volume decreases.

8. True or False: As tube diameter increases, flow volume increases.

9. True or False: As tube diameter decreases, flow volume decreases.

10. True or False: As tube length decreases, flow volume increases.

11. True or False: As tube length increases, flow volume decreases.

12. True or False: As fluid viscosity increases, flow volume decreases.

13. True or False: As fluid viscosity decreases, flow volume increases.

14. True or False: According to Poiseuille's law, tube radius has the greatest effect on flow volume.

15. True or False: Overall flow resistance may be increased by increasing fluid viscosity, increasing tube length and/or decreasing tube radius.

16. True or False: A change in tube radius will have the greatest effect on overall flow resistance.

BOARD REVIEW QUESTIONS - Section 6A

1. All of the following affect flow volume except:
   a. pressure gradient
   b. tube radius
   c. tube length
   d. flow direction

2. Which of the following varies directly with flow volume?
   a. pressure gradient
   b. tube length
   c. fluid viscosity
   d. fluid direction

3. According to Poiseuille's law, which of the following varies directly with flow volume?
   a. tube diameter
   b. tube length
   c. fluid viscosity
   d. fluid direction

4. According to Poiseuille's law, which of the following varies inversely with flow volume?
   a. pressure gradient
   b. tube diameter
   c. tube length
   d. fluid direction

5. According to Poiseuille's law, which of the following varies inversely with flow volume?
   a. pressure gradient
   b. tube diameter
   c. fluid viscosity
   d. fluid direction

6. As the pressure gradient increases, flow volume:
   a. increases
   b. decreases
   c. varies
   d. cannot be predicted

7. As tube diameter increases, flow volume:
   a. increases
   b. decreases
   c. varies
   d. cannot be predicted

8. As fluid viscosity increases, flow volume:
    a. increases
    b. decreases
    c. varies
    d. cannot be predicted

9. According to Poiseuille's law, which of the following has the greatest effect on flow volume?
    a. pressure gradient
    b. tube diameter
    c. tube length
    d. fluid viscosity

10. All of the following will increase overall flow resistance in a tube except:
    a. decrease tube radius
    b. increase fluid viscosity
    c. increase tube length
    d. change in flow direction

11. Which of the following will have the greatest effect on overall flow resistance?
    a. fluid viscosity
    b. tube radius
    c. tube length
    d. pressure gradient

ANSWERS - Section 6A

Review practice answers

1. True
2. directly
3. directly
4. True
5. True
6. True
7. True
8. True
9. True
10. True
11. True
12. True
13. True
14. True
15. True
16. True

Board review answers

1. d
2. a
3. b
4. c
5. c
6. a
7. a
8. b
9. b
10. d
11. b

2. LAMINAR FLOW

3. DISTURBED FLOW

There are five types of steady flow:

    inlet
    laminar
    parabolic
    disturbed
    turbulent

Inlet flow: In inlet (plug) flow all velocities are equal at all radical distances from the center of the tube. Inlet flow is usually located at the entrance of a great vessel.

Laminar flow: Laminar flow is present when the fluid particle motion becomes smooth and parallel to each other. Fully developed laminar flow becomes parabolic in shape.

Disturbed flow: Disturbed flow occurs at an area of stenosis or vessel bifurcation where the fluid particles still flow in a forward direction but have been disturbed.

Inlet, parabolic and disturbed flow are types of laminar flow.

Turbulent flow: Turbulent flow occurs when the fluid particles move in multiple directions and different velocities and is considered abnormal flow. Vortices (fluid with whirling or circular motion) or eddies (small circular currents) may develop where the blood flow becomes turbulent. Turbulent flow's net direction is forward. Reynolds number predicts the onset of turbulent flow.

Reynolds number (Re) = flow speed x tube radius x fluid density / fluid viscosity

In cardiovascular applications, fluid density and fluid viscosity are constant and therefore the flow speed (velocity) and tube diameter (radius) determine when turbulent flow will develop. A Reynolds number greater than 2000 indicates the development of turbulent flow. When turbulence is present, the pressure gradient increases rapidly due to the dissipation of hydraulic energy into turbulent flow.

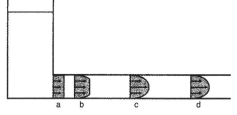

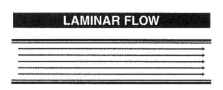

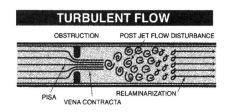

CHAPTER 6 (UNIT SIX) - PRINCIPLES OF CARDIAC HEMODYNAMICS

REVIEW PRACTICE - Section 6A

1. The five types of steady flow are: 1._____, 2._____, 3._____, 4._____ and 5._____.

2. In _____ flow, all velocities are equal at all radical distances from the center of the tube.

3. True or False: Inlet flow is also called plug flow.

4. In _____ flow, fluid particles move smoothly and are parallel to one another and is considered normal flow.

5. True or False: Fully developed laminar flow becomes parabolic in shape.

6. _____ flow occurs at areas of stenosis or vessel bifurcation where the fluid particles still flow in a forward direction but have been disturbed.

7. True or False: Inlet, parabolic and disturbed flow are all types of laminar flow.

8. _____ flow is present when fluid particles move in multiple directions and velocities with vortices possibly being created.

9. True or False: Turbulent flow is considered abnormal flow.

10. True or False: Reynolds number predicts when turbulent flow will occur.

11. For cardiovascular applications, flow _____ and vessel _____ have the greatest influence on when turbulent flow will develop.

12. A Reynolds number that exceeds _____ indicates the development of turbulent flow.

13. True or False: When turbulent flow is present, the pressure gradient increases rapidly due to the dissipation of hydraulic energy into turbulent flow, friction and heat energy.

BOARD REVIEW QUESTIONS - Section 6A

1. Flow in which fluid layers slide over each other in a smooth, orderly manner is:
   a. laminar
   b. turbulent
   c. Reynolds
   d. abnormal

2. Laminar flow is considered:
   a. abnormal
   b. normal
   c. varied
   d. turbulent

3. The type of flow where all velocities are equal at all radical distances from the center of the tube is:
   a. inlet
   b. disturbed
   c. turbulent
   d. parabolic

4. Inlet flow is also called:
   a. disturbed
   b. turbulent
   c. parabolic
   d. plug

5. The type of flow where the fluid particles move smoothly and are parallel to one another is:
   a. turbulent
   b. laminar
   c. abnormal
   d. eddy

6. The type of flow that may develop at an area of stenosis or vessel bifurcation is:
   a. inlet
   b. outlet
   c. disturbed
   d. vortice

7. All of the following are types of laminar flow except:
   a. inlet
   b. parabolic
   c. disturbed
   d. turbulent

CHAPTER 6 (UNIT SIX) - PRINCIPLES OF CARDIAC HEMODYNAMICS

8. The type of flow present when fluid particles move in multiple directions and velocities is:
   a. inlet
   b. laminar
   c. turbulent
   d. disturbed

9. Turbulent flow is considered:
   a. normal
   b. abnormal
   c. inlet
   d. outlet

10. The number that may be used to predict when turbulent flow will occur is:
   a. Bernoulli
   b. Doppler
   c. Reynolds
   d. Gorlin

11. For cardiovascular applications which of the following have the greatest effect on when turbulent flow will occur?
   a. flow speed, fluid viscosity
   b. fluid viscosity, fluid density
   c. flow speed, tube diameter
   d. fluid viscosity, tube diameter

ANSWERS - Section 6A

Review practice answers

1. inlet, laminar, parabolic, disturbed, turbulent
2. inlet
3. True
4. laminar
5. True
6. disturbed
7. True
8. turbulent
9. True
10. True
11. speed (velocity), diameter (radius)
12. 2000
13. True

Board review answers

1. a
2. b
3. a
4. d
5. b
6. c
7. d
8. c
9. b
10. c
11. c

4. RELATIONSHIPS BETWEEN PRESSURE AND VELOCITY

Bernoulli Equation

Bernoulli's principle states that there will be an increase in kinetic energy with a decrease in pressure at the site of an obstruction to flow. This is based on the conservation of energy principle which describes the relationship between potential (pressure) energy, kinetic energy and gravitational energy. If one of these energies changes, there will be a change in the other energies to maintain the same level of total energy.

The Bernoulli equation demonstrates that velocity and pressure are inversely related. As velocity increases, for example at the site of a stenosis, the pressure drops. As velocity decreases distal to the stenosis the pressure increases. The Bernoulli equation is utilized clinically to predict this pressure drop (gradient) between two chambers.

$$P_1 - P_2 = \frac{1}{2}\rho(v_2^2 - v_1^2) + \rho\int_1^2 \frac{dv}{dt}\,ds + R(\mu, v)$$

$$\text{Convective Acceleration} \qquad \text{Flow Acceleration} \qquad \text{Viscous Friction}$$

$$\Delta P = \frac{1}{2}\rho(v_2^2 - v_1^2) \quad \text{[Short acceleration, brief contact with walls]}$$

$$\Delta P = 4(v_2^2 - v_1^2) \quad \text{[Pressure in mmHg velocity in m/sec]}$$

$$\Delta P = 4v_2^2 \quad [v_1 << v_2]$$

Simplified Bernoulli Equation

In clinical imaging ultrasound, proximal velocity (V_1), flow acceleration and viscous friction are ignored. The relationship between pressure and velocity is then expressed as: $P1 - P2 = 4 \times (V_2)^2$

The clinical pitfalls of utilizing the simplified Bernoulli equation $4 \times (V_2)^2$, which ignores the proximal velocity (V_1), flow acceleration and viscous friction includes:

If the proximal velocity (V_1) is greater than 1.0 m/s the pressure gradient may be overestimated.

In tunnel like stenosis (coarctation, certain types of prosthetic heart valves) or stenosis in a series (e.g. coronary artery disease), the predicted pressure gradient using the simplified Bernoulli equation will be too low due to ignoring viscous friction.

Cardiac Doppler Pressure Gradient

Factors that may cause a discrepancy between a cardiac Doppler pressure gradient derived by the Bernoulli equation and a cardiac catheterization derived pressure gradient include:

Comparison of the catheterization peak to peak pressure gradient with the Doppler peak pressure gradient.

Failure to consider the proximal velocity (V_1) may lead to an overestimation of the pressure gradient.

The pressure recovery phenomenon may cause an overestimation.

Recording the wrong jet (e.g. mitral regurgitation instead of the aortic stenosis jet) may lead to an overestimation.

Failure to record the peak velocity may cause an underestimation of the true pressure gradient.

Changing physiologic conditions may lead to an underestimation.

REVIEW PRACTICE - Section 6A

1. True or False: There will be an decrease in potential (pressure) energy with an increase in kinetic energy at the site of a flow obstruction.

2. True or False: A pressure drop or gradient may be predicted by the Bernoulli equation.

3. True or False: In clinical imaging ultrasound, proximal velocity (V_1), flow acceleration and viscous friction of the Bernoulli equation are ignored.

4. The formula used in clinical imaging ultrasound to predict the pressure drop (gradient) across an obstruction is 4 x _____.

5. True or False: The pitfalls of the simplified Bernoulli equation 4 x $(V_2)\approx$ include a proximal velocity of greater than 1.0 m/s, stenosis in series, and long, tunnel like stenosis.

Determine the pressure gradient for the following velocities using the simplified Bernoulli equation:

6. 1.0 m/s:_____ mm Hg

7. 2.0 m/s:_____ mm Hg

8. 3.0 m/s:_____ mm Hg

9. 4.0 m/s:_____ mm Hg

10. 5.0 m/s:_____ mm Hg

11. 6.0 m/s:_____ mm Hg

Determine the pressure gradient from the following velocities using the lengthened Bernoulli equation: 4 x $(V_2^2 - V_1^2)$:

12. $V_2 = 3.0$ m/s; $V_1 = 1.0$ m/s:_____ mm Hg

13. $V_2 = 4.0$ m/s; $V_1 = 2.0$ m/s:_____ mm Hg

14. $V_2 = 6.0$ m/s; $V_1 = 3.0$ m/s:_____ mm Hg

15. Check the following if a possible reason for creating a discrepancy between a Doppler derived pressure gradient and a cardiac catheterization pressure gradient:

_____ comparison of the cardiac catheterization peak to peak gradient to the Doppler peak pressure gradient

_____ failure to consider the proximal velocity (V_1)

_____ pressure recovery phenomenon

_____ recording the wrong jet

_____ failure to record the peak velocity

_____ changing physiologic conditions

Tell if the following will cause a cardiac Doppler underestimation or overestimation of the cardiac catheterization pressure gradient:

16. _____comparing the cardiac catheterization peak to peak pressure gradient to the cardiac Doppler peak pressure gradient

17. _____ failure to consider the proximal velocity

18. _____ pressure recovery phenomenon

19. _____ recording of the wrong jet (mitral regurgitation jet instead of the aortic stenosis jet)

20. _____ failure to record the maximum peak velocity

21. _____ changing physiologic conditions

CHAPTER 6 (UNIT SIX) - PRINCIPLES OF CARDIAC HEMODYNAMICS

BOARD REVIEW QUESTIONS - Section 6A

1. The principle that suggests that there will be an increase in kinetic energy with a decrease in pressure at the site of an obstruction is:
   a. Doppler
   b. Bernoulli
   c. Gorlin
   d. Ohm

2. The Bernoulli equation predicts a (the):
   a. fluid velocity
   b. pressure gradient
   c. kinetic energy
   d. fluid direction

3. In clinical imaging ultrasound, all of the following components of the Bernoulli equation are ignored except:
   a. $(V_2)^2$
   b. viscous friction
   c. flow acceleration
   d. proximal velocity

4. The simplified Bernoulli equation is:
   a. $4 \times (V_2)^2$
   b. CSA x VTI
   c. EDV - ESV
   d. CO x HR

5. All of the following are considered pitfalls of the simplified Bernoulli equation except:
   a. proximal velocity greater than 1.0 m/s
   b. short, discrete stenosis
   c. stenosis in a series
   d. pressure recovery

6. The pressure gradient between the right ventricle and the right atrium in a patient with a tricuspid regurgitation velocity of 3.0 m/s is:
   a. 3 mm Hg
   b. 9 mm Hg
   c. 36 mm Hg
   d. 46 mm Hg

CHAPTER 6 (UNIT SIX) - PRINCIPLES OF CARDIAC HEMODYNAMICS

7. The peak aortic valve velocity in a patient with valvular aortic stenosis is determined to be 5.0 m/s. The left ventricular outflow tract velocity is 2.0 m/s. The peak pressure gradient utilizing the lengthened Bernoulli equation is:
   a. 5 mm Hg
   b. 25 mm Hg
   c. 84 mm Hg
   d. 100 mm Hg

8. All of the following are possible clincal pitfalls when using the simplified Bernoulli equation of $4 \times (V_2)^2$ except:
   a. ignoring the V_1 velocity
   b. tunnel like stenosis
   c. stenosis in a series
   d. ignoring convective acceleration

9. All of the following may cause a discrepancy between a Doppler derived pressure gradient and a cardiac catheterization derived presure gradient, except:
   a. comparison of the cardiac catheterization peak to peak pressure gradient with the Doppler peak pressure gradient
   b. failure to consider the proximal velocity
   c. pressure recovery phenomenon
   d. intercepting blood flow at 0 degrees

ANSWERS - Section 6A

Review practice answers

1. True
2. True
3. True
4. $(V_2)^2$
5. True
6. 4 mm Hg
7. 16 mm Hg
8. 36 mm Hg
9. 64 mm Hg
10. 100 mm Hg
11. 144 mm Hg
12. 32 mm Hg
13. 48 mm Hg
14. 108 mm Hg
15. all
16. overestimation
17. overestimation
18. overestimation
19. overestimation
20. underestimation
21. underestimation

Board review answers

1. b
2. b
3. a
4. a
5. b
6. c
7. c
8. d
9. d

SECTION 6B
Effects of Abnormal Pressures and Loading

1. HEART FAILURE AND SHOCK

Heart failure: The inability of the heart to meet the metabolic demands of the body.
Causes: Myocardial dysfunction (e.g. myocardial infarction)
              Pressure overload (e.g. aortic stenosis)
              Volume overload (e.g. mitral regurgitation)
              Diastolic dysfunction (e.g. amyloidosis)
              Increased metabolic demands (e.g. anemia)

Although heart failure may originate in the right ventricle, it usually begins with the left ventricle. Since the ventricles are connected in series, failure of one ventricle will eventually lead to biventricular failure.

As the left ventricle fails, stimulation of the baroreceptors in the aorta and reflex stimulation of the sympathetic nervous system occurs. This leads to vasoconstriction of the veins, thus increasing venous return and vasoconstriction of the arteries, leading to an increase in systemic blood pressure. Myocardial contractility responds by increasing, and the heart rate also increases.

The kidneys respond by releasing renin, which will promote further vasoconstriction and fluid retention. This will continue to increase blood pressure, blood volume and venous return.

The failing left ventricle cannot adequately respond to the compensatory mechanisms and these compensatory mechanisms eventually leads to an increase in left ventricular myocardial oxygen demand, blood volume and pressure. This increased left ventricular pressure is reflected back to the pulmonary vasculature leading to pulmonary congestion. This is why it is referred to as congestive heart failure. The patient complains of dyspnea due to the pulmonary congestion. Eventually the right ventricle will fail due to the increase in pulmonary pressures and will be manifested by systemic changes such as peripheral edema and hepatomegaly.

The treatment for congestive heart failure is to remove the underlying etiology, such as coronary artery bypass for myocardial ischemia. Drug treatment for congestive heart failure may include positive inotropes, vasodilators and diuretics.

CARDIOGENIC SHOCK

Cardiogenic shock is shock resulting from failure to maintain blood supply to the circulatory system and tissues due to inadequate cardiac output. Cardiogenic shock may be seen in patients with acute myocardial infarction, end-stage cardiomyopathy, or a mechanical defect such as flail valve leaflet, acquired ventricular septal defect or cardiac tamponade.

2. VALVULAR STENOSIS

Aortic/Pulmonic: Pressure overload of ventricle results initially with hypertrophy developing first, then dilatation when ventricular failure occurs.

Mitral/Tricuspid: Pressure overload of the atrium with atrial dilatation with the potential for pressure to be "reflected back" into respective venous system.

3. VALVULAR REGURGITATION

Aortic/Pulmonic: Volume overload of the ventricle with dilatation initially, followed by ventricular dilatation and hypertrophy long term.

Mitral/Tricuspid: Volume overload of the atrium with atrial dilatation coupled with ventricular dilatation long term.

4. SHUNTS

Atrial septal defect: Volume overload of the right atrium, right ventricle and pulmonary circulation.

Ventricular septal defect: Volume overload of the pulmonary circulation, left atrium and left ventricle.

Patent ductus arteriosus: Volume overload of the pulmonary system, left atrium and left ventricle.

5. PULMONARY DISEASE

Intrinsic pulmonary disease is a pressure overload of the right ventricle with initial hypertrophy followed long term by right ventricular dilatation. Right heart failure due to intrinsic pulmonary disease is called cor pulmonale.

6. PERICARDIAL DISEASE

Cardiac tamponade results in equalization of diastolic pressures due to an increase in intrapericardial pressure. This increase in intrapericardial pressure reduces diastolic ventricular filling and leads to a decrease in stroke volume and cardiac output and diastolic collapse of the cardiac chamber walls.

Constrictive pericarditis is the abnormal thickening of the pericardium resulting in a reduction of the elastic properties of the pericardium. This stiffening of the pericardium will eventually reduce ventricular diastolic filling, stroke volume and cardiac output.

7. CARDIOMYOPATHIES

Hypertrophic cardiomyopathy is initially a pressure overload of the left ventricle. Dilated cardiomyopathy results initially in a volume overload of the ventricles and atria. Restrictive cardiomyopathy results in an increase in ventricular and atrial diastolic pressures.

REVIEW PRACTICE - Section 6A

1. Congestive _____ _____ is the inability of the heart to meet the metabolic demands of the body.

2. True or False: A possible cause for congestive heart failure is myocardial damage as what may occur in coronary artery disease.

3. True or False: A possible cause of congestive heart failure is pressure overload as what may occur in valvular aortic stenosis.

4. True or False: A possible cause of congestive heart failure is volume overload such as that seen in significant chronic mitral regurgitation.

5. True or False: A possible cause of congestive heart failure is diastolic dysfunction such as that may be seen in advanced cardiac amyloidosis.

6. True or False: A possible cause of congestive heart failure is increased metabolic demands such as severe anemia, thyrotoxicosis, pregnancy, fever or sepsis.

7. _____ shock results in shock from failure of the heart to maintain adequate cardiac output.

Tell whether the following are initially considered a pressure overload or volume overload:

8. Aortic stenosis: Pressure/Volume

9. Pulmonic stenosis: Pressure/Volume

10. Mitral stenosis   Pressure/Volume

11. Tricuspid stenosis: Pressure/Volume

12. Aortic regurgitation: Pressure/Volume

13. Pulmonary regurgitation: Pressure/Volume

14. Mitral regurgitation: Pressure/Volume

15. Tricuspid regurgitation Pressure/Volume

Tell whether the following shunts are a volume or pressure overload:

16. Atrial septal defect: Volume/Pressure

17. Ventricular septal defect: Volume/Pressure

18. Patent ductus arteriosus: Volume/Pressure

19. True or False: Intrinsic pulmonary disease may first lead to right ventricular hypertrophy and eventually to right ventricular dilatation.

20. True or False: Cardiac tamponade leads to an increase in intrapericardial pressures, an equalization of intracardiac diastolic pressures, and a decrease in diastolic filling, stroke volume and cardiac output.

21. True or False: Constrictive pericarditis is the thickening of the pericardium which will lead to impaired ventricular diastolic filling, stroke volume and cardiac output.

22. Hypertrophic cardiomyopathy is a pressure?/volume? overload of the left ventricle.

23. Dilated cardiomyopathy results initially in a pressure?/volume? overload.

24. True or False: Restrictive cardiomyopathy results in an increase in ventricular and atrial diastolic pressures.

BOARD REVIEW QUESTIONS - Section 6B

1. The inability of the heart to meet the metabolic demands of the body is:
    a. congestive heart failure
    b. cardiomyopathy
    c. stenosis
    d. regurgitation

2. All of the following may be a cause of congestive heart failure except:
    a. aortic dilatation
    b. myocardial damage
    c. pressure/volume overload
    d. diastolic dysfunction

3. Aortic stenosis initially results in a:
    a. ventricular pressure overload
    b. ventricular volume overload
    c. atrial volume overload
    d. pulmonary hypertension

4. Pulmonary stenosis initially results in a:
    a. ventricular pressure overload
    b. ventricular volume overload
    c. atrial volume overload
    d. pulmonary hypertension

5. Mitral stenosis initially results in a:
    a. pressure overload of the left ventricle
    b. volume overload of the left ventricle
    c. pressure overload of the left atrium
    d. systemic hypertension

6. Tricuspid stenosis initially results in a:
    a. ventricular volume overload
    b. ventricular pressure overload
    c. right atrial pressure overload
    d. pulmonary hypertension

7. Aortic regurgitation initially results in a:
    a. ventricular pressure overload
    b. ventricular volume overload
    c. atrial hypertrophy
    d. atrial dilatation

8. Pulmonary regurgitation initially results in a:
    a. ventricular volume overload
    b. ventricular pressure overload
    c. atrial volume overload
    d. pulmonary hypertension

9. Mitral regurgitation initially results in a:
    a. pressure overload of the left ventricle
    b. volume overload of the left heart
    c. volume overload of the right heart
    d. systemic hypertension

10. Tricuspid regurgitation initially results in a:
    a. ventricular/atrial pressure overload
    b. volume overload of the right heart
    c. pulmonary hypertension
    d. systemic hypertension

11. An atrial septal defect will result in a volume overload of all of the following except:
    a. right atrium
    b. left atrium
    c. right ventricle
    d. main pulmonary artery

12. A ventricular septal defect will result in a volume overload of all of the following except:
    a. left atrium
    b. right ventricle
    c. pulmonary veins
    d. left ventricle

13. A patent ductus arteriosus will result in a volume overload of all of the following except:
    a. left atrium
    b. left ventricle
    c. pulmonary veins
    d. right ventricle

14. Intrinsic pulmonary disease may result in:
    a. left atrial dilatation
    b. carcinoid
    c. Eisenmenger's
    d. cor pulmonale

15. Cardiac tamponade may result in all of the following except:
    a. diastolic equalization of intracardiac pressures
    b. systolic equalization of intracardiac pressures
    c. diastolic collapse of the right atrium
    d. inferior vena cava plethora

16. Constrictive pericarditis may result in all of the following except:
    a. abnormal thickening of the pericardium
    b. decreased ventricular diastolic filling
    c. decreased stroke volume
    d. ventricular volume overload

17. Hypertrophic cardiomyopathy initially results in a:
    a. left ventricular pressure overload
    b. right ventricular pressure overload
    c. left atrial pressure overload
    d. right atrial pressure overload

18. Dilated cardiomyopathy initially results in a:
    a. volume overload of the ventricles/atria
    b. pressure overload of the ventricles/atria
    c. pulmonary hypertension
    d. systemic hypertension

ANSWERS - Section 6B

Review practice answers

1. heart failure
2. True
3. True
4. True
5. True
6. True
7. cardiogenic
8. pressure
9. pressure
10. pressure
11. pressure
12. volume
13. volume
14. volume
15. volume
16. volume
17. volume
18. volume
19. True
20. True
21. True
22. pressure
23. volume
24. True

Board review answers

1.	a	14.	d
2.	a	15.	b
3.	a	16.	d
4.	a	17.	a
5.	c	18.	a
6.	c		
7.	b		
8.	a		
9.	b		
10.	b		
11.	b		
12.	b		
13.	d		

CHAPTER 6 (UNIT SIX) - PRINCIPLES OF CARDIAC HEMODYNAMICS

APPENDICES

A. WIGGER'S DIAGRAM

B. CARDIOVASCULAR PRINCIPLES AT A GLANCE

C. CARDIOVASCULAR PRINCIPLES 500

D. SOCIETIES

APPENDIX A

APPENDIX A
WIGGER'S DIAGRAM

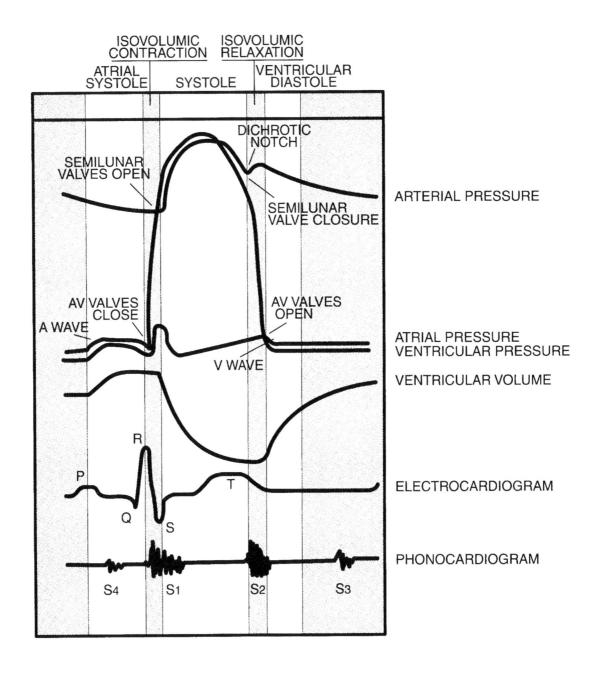

APPENDIX B
CARDIOVASCULAR PRINCIPLES AT A GLANCE

ANATOMY of the HEART

The heart is a pump with two receiving chambers (atria) and two pumping chambers (ventricles) that moves blood in a series.

ATRIA

The right atrium receives deoxygenated blood from the superior vena, inferior vena cava and coronary sinus during ventricular systole and delivers this blood to the right ventricle during ventricular diastole.

The right atrium is composed of two chambers: the principal cavity (sinus venosus) and the atrial appendage.

In the right atrium there are important anatomical structures: the eustachian valve, network of Chiari, thebesian valve and the pectinate muscles.

The eustachian valve guards the opening of the inferior vena cava.

The fenestrated portion of the eustachian valve is the network of Chiari.

The thebesian valve guards the opening of the coronary sinus.

The pectinate muscles are located along the free wall and in the atrial appendage of the right atrium.

The sulcus terminalis is a posterior external ridge that extends from the superior vena cava to the inferior vena cava.

The crista terminalis is the internal ridge that corresponds to the sulcus terminalis.

The aorta lies in close proximity to the right atrium (torus aorticus) and sinus of Valsalva aneurysm may rupture into the right atrium.

The left atrium receives oxygenated blood from the four pulmonary veins during ventricular systole and delivers this blood to the left ventricle during ventricular diastole.

The left atrium consists of two sections: the principal cavity and the atrial appendage.

Pectinate muscles striate the free wall and atrial appendage of the left atrium.

The interatrial septum divides the two atria into relatively equal halves.

The central portion of the interatrial septum is called the foramen ovale in the fetus and the fossa ovalis in the adult.

The ridge around the fossa ovalis is called the limbus of the fossa ovalis and may be visualized anatomically from the right atrium.

Approximately 25% of adults have a patent foramen ovale.

APPENDIX B

VENTRICLES

The ventricles contain trabeculae carneae, papillary muscles and chordae tendineae.

The right ventricle pumps deoxygenated blood to the lungs via the pulmonary artery during ventricular systole.

The right ventricle is thin walled as compared to the left ventricle because the right ventricle pumps blood against a low resistance: the lungs.

The right ventricle is the most anterior cardiac structure and appears triangular in shape externally.

The right ventricle has an inflow tract, apex and outflow tract.

The right ventricle has three papillary muscle sets: anterior, posterior and medial (conal).

The right ventricular apex is heavily trabeculated.

The area of the right ventricle immediately beneath the pulmonic valve is called the infundibulum.

The right ventricle has three important muscle bands: moderator band, septal band and the crista supraventricularis.

The left ventricle is a thick muscular chamber which pumps oxygenated blood into the high resistance systemic circulation during ventricular systole.

The two papillary muscle sets of the left ventricle are called the anterolateral and posteromedial.

The left ventricle forms the cardiac apex.

The normal left ventricle is considered a prolate ellipse.

The interventricular septum separates the right ventricle from the left ventricle. It has two components: the muscular septum and membranous septum.

The muscular septum has three regions: inlet, trabecular and outlet.

In the normal heart the interventricular septum is concave to the left ventricle and convex to the right ventricle because left ventricular pressures are higher than right ventricular pressures.

CARDIAC VALVES

The left heart atrioventricular valve is the mitral valve with two leaflets (anterior and posterior) and two commissures (lateral and medial).

The posterior mitral valve has three scallops: lateral, medial and middle (largest).

The right heart atrioventricular valve is the tricuspid valve with three leaflets called the anterior (largest), medial (septal) and posterior (smallest).

The left heart semilunar valve is the aortic valve composed of three cusps (right, left and non-coronary), commissures, sinuses of Valsalva and the nodules of Arantii.

The most common acyanotic congenital heart defect in the adult population is the bicuspid aortic valve.

The right heart semilunar valve is the pulmonic valve composed of three cusps (right, left and anterior), commissures, sinuses and nodules of Atlantii.

ARTERIAL-VENOUS SYSTEM

The aorta carries oxygenated blood to the body and its sections include the aortic annulus, sinotubular junction, ascending aorta, aortic (transverse) arch, descending thoracic aorta and abdominal aorta.

The aortic arch gives off three vessels: brachiocephalic (innominate) artery, left common carotid artery and left subclavian artery.

The aortic isthmus is the small segment of the aorta located between the end of the left subclavian artery and the insertion of the ligamentum arteriosum (ductus arteriosus).

The right coronary artery originates from the right sinus of Valsalva proceeds anteriorly and posteriorly between the right atrium and right ventricle in the coronary sulcus. In a majority of humans (67%) the right coronary artery provides the posterior descending artery (right dominant) which supplies oxygenated blood to the inferior surface of the heart.

The right coronary artery provides oxygenated blood to the right atrium, sinoatrial node, atrioventricular node, right ventricle, inferior wall of the left ventricle and inferior interventricular septum.

The left coronary artery originates from the left sinus of Valsalva and bifurcates from the left main into the left anterior descending coronary artery and left circumflex coronary artery.

The left anterior descending coronary artery provides oxygenated blood to the anterior interventricular septum, anterior wall of the left ventricle and cardiac apex.

The left circumflex coronary artery provides oxygenated blood to the anterolateral, lateral and inferolateral walls of the left ventricle.

The coronary sinus, which has the lowest oxygen saturation content of any vessel in the body (60%), collects the hearts' deoxygenated blood and is made up of three tributaries: great cardiac vein, middle cardiac vein and the small cardiac vein.

The great cardiac vein drains the left anterior descending and left circumflex coronary arteries.

The middle cardiac vein drains the posterior descending coronary artery.

The small cardiac vein drains the right coronary artery.

The pulmonary artery connects the right ventricle to the lungs and is the only artery in the body to carry deoxygenated blood.

The four pulmonary veins carry oxygenated blood to the left atrium thus are the only veins in the body to carry oxygenated blood.

CARDIAC CONDUCTION SYSTEM

The cardiac conduction system consists of the sinoatrial (SA) node, internodal pathways (Bachmann's most developed), bundle of His, right and left bundle branches and the Purkinje fibers.

Ventricular depolarization occurs from endocardium to epicardium and the heart contracts from apex to base.

APPENDIX B

LAYERS

The heart consists of three layers: the inner layer called the endocardium, the thick muscular layer called the myocardium and the thin outer layer called the epicardium (visceral pericardium).

The heart lies in a protective sac called the pericardium The pericardium consists of two layers. The external layer called the fibrous (parietal) pericardium and a thin, inner membrane which lines the fibrous (parietal) pericardium called the parietal serous pericardium.

The pericardial space lies between the parietal serous pericardium and the epicardium and normally contains up to 50 cc of fluid.

Adipose tissue is fitted between the epicardium and myocardium.

The pericardial-pulmonary vein interface creates a potential space called the oblique sinus.

The pericardial-great vessel interface creates a potential space called the transverse sinus.

RELATIONAL ANATOMY

The heart lies behind the sternum in the mediastinal cavity with the tip of the heart called the cardiac apex and the upper portion called the base.

Externally the crux of the heart is the point where the coronary sinus and the posterior descending coronary artery meet externally and where the atrioventricular valves and the septa meet internally.

The pulmonary valve lies superior, anterior and to the left of the aortic valve.

Compared to the mitral valve, the tricuspid valve is inserted closer to the cardiac apex.

During ventricular systole the heart moves downward (base to apex), twists counterclockwise and moves anteriorly.

BASIC EMBRYOLOGY

The heart tube appears by week three and is fully developed by week seven.

The heart is the first organ to be completely formed in the fetus.

The heart tube loops anteriorly and rightward.

Cardiac septation occurs between days 27 and 37.

The seven regions of the heart tube are the: sinus venosus, primitive atria, atrioventricular canal, primitive ventricle, bulbus cordis, truncus arteriosus and the aortic sac and arches.

The sinus venosus contributes to the development of the vena cava, coronary sinus and the posterior wall of the atria.

The primitive atria is divided equally by the interatrial septum which is formed by the septum primum and septum secundum.

The atrioventricular canal is the orifice that lies between the primitive atria and primitive ventricle. It is eventually divided into the atrioventricular orifices by the endocardial cushions. The endocardial cushions also contribute to the formation of the anterior mitral valve, septal tricuspid valve and interventricular septum.

The primitive ventricle is a morphologic left ventricle.

APPENDIX B

The bulbus cordis contributes to the formation of the right ventricle, outflow tracts and the great vessel trunks.

The truncus arteriosus contributes to the formation of the great vessel roots.

The third aortic arch contributes to the formation of the internal carotid artery. The fourth aortic arch becomes the aortic arch. The sixth aortic arch develops into the right and left pulmonary arteries and the ductus arteriosus.

FETAL and POSTNATAL CIRCULATION

The oxygenated blood from the placenta enters the umbilical vein is delivered to the inferior vena cava after bypassing the liver via the ductus venosus into the right atrium.

Two thirds of the blood that enters the right atrium via the inferior vena cava is deflected by the eustachian valve through the foramen ovale into the left atrium where it travels out the aorta.

One third of the blood returned by the inferior vena cava mixes in the right atrium with the deoxygenated blood returned from the upper part of the fetus. This blood then travels to the right ventricle out the pulmonary artery. Since the lungs are deflated, most of this blood is shunted through the ductus arteriosus to the descending thoracic aorta to the umbilical arteries and back to the placenta.

After birth the pulmonary vascular resistance drops while left heart pressures rise, the foramen ovale closes and becomes the fossa ovalis, the ductus arteriosus closes and becomes the ligamentum arteriosum and the ductus venosus closes to become the ligamentum venosum.

CONGENITAL DEFECTS

The types of atrial septal defects include the ostium secundum, ostium primum, sinus venosus and the coronary sinus.

The ostium secundum atrial septal defect involves the central portion of the interatrial septum and is associated with mitral valve prolapse.

The ostium primum atrial septal defect involves the inferior portion of the interatrial septum and is associated with cleft mitral valve.

The sinus venosus atrial septal defect affects the superior portion of the atrial septum and is associated with partial anomalous pulmonary venous return.

The four types of ventricular septal defects are the perimembranous, muscular (trabecular), inlet (posterior, AV canal type) and outlet (subpulmonic, supracristal).

The perimembranous defect is located beneath the aortic valve in the left ventricular outflow tract.

The muscular (trabecular) defect may be located throughout the muscular septum and may be multiple.

The inlet (posterior, AV canal type) defect is located posteriorly beneath the posterior leaflet of the tricuspid valve.

The outlet (subpulmonic, supracristal) defect is located beneath the pulmonary valve in the right ventricular outflow tract.

Coarctation is an abnormal narrowing of the descending thoracic aorta and is commonly associated with bicuspid aortic valve.

Tetralogy of Fallot consists of four lesions: malalignment ventricular septal defect, subpulmonic stenosis, overriding aorta and right ventricular hypertrophy.

d-transposition of the great vessels occurs when the aorta originates from the right ventricle and the pulmonary artery originates from the left ventricle.

l-transposition of the great vessels is present when there is ventricular inversion and the aorta arises from the morphologic right ventricle and the pulmonary artery originates from the morphologic left ventricle.

Truncus arteriosus is present when one great artery (aorta) gives rise to the coronary arteries, pulmonary artery and aortic arch. A malalignment ventricular septal defect is present.

Double outlet right ventricle occurs when the aorta and pulmonary artery both originate from the right ventricle. There is a malalignment ventricular septal defect present as well.

Persistent fetal circulation will occur if the pulmonary vascular resistance does not drop due to pulmonary hypertension after birth thus maintaining a right-to-left shunt through the foramen ovale and ductus arteriosus.

A patent ductus arteriosus is the communication between the pulmonary artery and aorta that persists after birth.

A complete atrioventricular septal defect includes an ostium primum atrial septal defect, inlet ventricular septal defect and a common atrioventricular valve.

A partial atrioventricular septal defect includes an ostium primum atrial septal defect and a cleft atrioventricular valve.

Ebstein's anomaly is the abnormal insertion of the tricuspid valve towards the cardiac apex with atrialization of the right ventricle.

Uhl's anomaly is the absence of right ventricular myocardial tissue.

Aortic stenosis may be supravalvular, valvular or subvalvular.

Pulmonic stenosis may be supravalvular, valvular or subvalvular.

Tricuspid atresia is characterized by the complete absence of the tricuspid valve resulting in a lack of communication between the right atrium and right ventricle with hypoplasia of the right ventricle.

Mitral atresia is characterized by the complete absence of the mitral valve resulting in a lack of communication between the left atrium and left ventricle with hypoplasia of the left ventricle.

Pulmonary atresia with intact interventricular septum is complete obstruction of the right ventricular outflow tract with an atretic pulmonary valve, an intact interventricular septum and variable hypoplasia of the right ventricle and tricuspid valve.

Cor triatriatum is characterized by a perforate membrane that partitions the left atrium.

Supravalvular mitral stenosis occurs when an obstructive ridge or stenosing ring is located just proximal to the mitral valve.

APPENDIX B

PROPAGATION of ELECTRICAL ACTIVITY

The electrical impulse normally travels from the sinoatrial (SA) node through the internodal pathways to the atrioventricular (AV) node where there is a slight pause of $1/10^{th}$ of a second. From the AV node the impulse travels to the bundle of His to the right and left bundle branches to the Purkinje fibers.

The normal duration of ventricular systole is 0.12 seconds.

The SA node has an inherent firing rate of between 60 - 100 times per minute, the His bundle a rate of between 40 to 60 times per minute and the Purkinje fibers between 20 to 40 times per minute.

The most developed of the internodal pathways is Bachmann's bundle which delivers the impulse to the left atrium.

The ventricles depolarize from endocardium to epicardium and contracts apex to base.

The left ventricle depolarizes slightly before the right ventricle.

The heart possesses the characteristics of automaticity, excitability, conductivity and contractility.

Automaticity means the heart can begin and maintain rhythmic activity without the aid of the nervous system.

Excitability means that the cardiac muscle can accept and respond to electrical impulses.

Conductivity infers that a cardiac cell is able to transfer an electrical impulse to a neighboring cardiac cell.

Contractility means the heart can respond to an electrical impulse by contracting.

EXCITATION-CONTRACTION COUPLING MECHANISM

The action potential curve depicts the electrical activity of a cardiac cell.

Phase 0 represents cardiac cell rapid depolarization.

Phase 1 represents a brief period of early rapid repolarization.

Phase 2 is the plateau phase and represents the influx of calcium causing actual mechanical contraction. This is the central component of the excitation-coupling mechanism and coincides with the ST segment of the electrocardiogram. Actual cardiac contraction occurs during this phase.

Phase 3 represents final rapid repolarization.

Phase 4 represents the resting phase.

Electrical activity slightly precedes mechanical activity.

The absolute refractory period refers to the period of time between phase 1 and 2 where the cardiac cell will not accept another electrical stimulus no matter how strong.

The relative refractory period refers to the period of time between phase 2 and 3 where the cardiac cell is able to respond to an electrical stimulus but only if the stimulus is very strong.

APPENDIX B

FRANK-STARLING LAW and PRELOAD

The Frank-Starling law of the heart states that the greater the stretch of the cardiac muscle cell, the greater the force of contraction. This is also referred to as the length-tension relationship where length refers to the stretch of the myocardial cell and tension refers to contraction.

Preload is the length to which a myocardial cell is stretched and may be measured clinically as the pulmonary wedge pressure, central venous pressure, ventricular end-diastolic pressure or ventricular end-diastolic volume.

According to the Frank-Starling law, as preload increases cardiac performance (e.g. stroke volume, cardiac output) will increase to a certain physiologic limit.

Atrioventricular valve regurgitation, semilunar valve regurgitation and congenital heart defect shunts (atrial septal defect, ventricular septal defect, patent ductus arteriosus) all increase preload.

An increase in preload is associated with chamber dilatation.

FORCE-VELOCITY RELATIONSHIP

Force refers to the load production that a myocardial fiber must produce.

Velocity refers to the rate of myocardial fiber shortening.

Afterload is the resistance the ventricles faces as it ejects blood.

As afterload (force) increases, cardiac performance (velocity or rate of myocardial fiber shortening) decreases.

Pathologies that increase afterload include ventricular outflow tract obstruction, systemic/pulmonary hypertension and coarctation of the aorta.

An increase in afterload is associated with chamber hypertrophy.

INTERVAL-STRENGTH RELATIONSHIP

Interval refers to the time period between heart beats.

Strength refers to ventricular contraction.

As the interval between heart beats increases, the strength of contraction will increase.

The best example of the interval strength relationship is the post-premature ventricular contraction (PVC) beat. The strength of ventricular contraction is increased after the compensatory pause of a PVC. This may be referred to as post extra-systolic potentiation.

VALVE OPENING and CLOSURE

The cardiac valves open and close due to a change in pressure.

The atrioventricular valves close at the onset of the QRS complex when ventricular pressure exceeds atrial pressure.

The atrioventricular valves open at the end of the T wave when ventricular pressure drops below atrial pressure.

Compared to the mitral valve, the tricuspid valve opens first and closes last.

The semilunar valves open when ventricular pressure exceeds arterial pressure in early ventricular systole.

The semilunar valves close when ventricular pressure drops below arterial pressure at the end of ventricular systole.

Compared to the aortic valve, the pulmonic valve opens first and closes last.

PHASES of the CARDIAC CYCLE

Ventricular diastole represents the period of time the ventricles are filling between the end of the T wave and the onset of the QRS complex.

Approximately 70% of diastolic filling occurs during early ventricular diastole.

Diastasis represents mid-diastole when there is equilibration of ventricular and atrial diastolic pressures with little filling of the ventricles occurring during this time period.

Atrial systole represents late diastolic filling due to atrial contraction as marked by the P wave of the electrocardiogram.

Atrial systole contributes approximately 30% to ventricular diastolic filling.

Isovolumic contraction (pre-ejection period) is an early systolic event occuring between atrioventricular valve closure and semilunar valve opening.

There is an increase in ventricular pressure with no change in ventricular volume during isovolumic contraction.

Ventricular systole occurs between the onset of the QRS complex to the end of the T wave and represents the time period where the ventricles are ejecting blood into the great arteries (systolic ejection period or time).

Ventricular volume is lowest at peak ventricular systole.

Isovolumic relaxation represents early ventricular diastole and begins with the closure of the semilunar valves to the opening of the atrioventricular valves.

During isovolumic relaxation the ventricular pressure is decreasing with no change in ventricular volume.

LEFT VENTRICULAR FUNCTION: INDICATORS and NORMAL VALUES

Stroke volume (EDV - ESV) is the amount of blood pumped out of the heart per beat. The normal range is 70 cc to 100 cc.

The cardiac Doppler formula which permits calculation of stroke volume is CSA x VTI where CSA is the cross-sectional area and VTI is the velocity time integral.

Cardiac output (SV x HR) is the amount of blood pumped out of the heart per minute. The normal range is 4 lpm to 8 lpm.

Cardiac index (CO/BSA) is cardiac output adjusted for body surface area. The normal range is 2.4 lpm/m≈ to 4.2 lpm/m≈.

Ejection fraction (SV/EDV x 100) is the percentage of blood pumped out of the heart per beat. The normal range is 62% ±12.

APPENDIX B

PULMONARY vs SYSTEMIC CIRCULATION

The pulmonary circulation consists of the right ventricle, main pulmonary artery and branches, pulmonary capillaries and the pulmonary veins.

The systemic circulation consists of the left ventricle, aorta, systemic and capillary network, cerebral veins, peripheral veins, abdominal veins and the vena cava.

When comparing the systemic circulation to the pulmonary circulation, the systemic circulation is/has: higher pressure, greater resistance, higher oxygen content, lower carbon dioxide content, thicker ventricular walls, higher overall volume, thicker vessel walls, blood traveling a greater distance and an equal stroke volume.

INTRACARDIAC PRESSURES (mm Hg)	OXYGEN SATURATION (%)
RA: 2 to 8	75
RV: 15 to 30/2 to 8	75
MPA: 15 to 30/4 to 12	75
LA: 2 to 12	98
LV: 100 to 140/3 to 12	98
Ao: 100 to 140/60 to 90	98

In the absence of RV inflow tract obstruction, the RA pressure is equal to the right ventricular diastolic pressure.

In the absence of right ventricular outflow tract obstruction, the RV systolic pressure equals the systolic pulmonary artery pressure.

The PA end-diastolic pressure reflects LA pressure and LV end-diastolic pressure. (pulmonary wedge pressure)

In the absence of left ventricular outflow tract obstruction, the aortic systolic pressure equals the left ventricular systolic pressure.

In normals, the greatest pressure difference in the heart exists between the left atrium and left ventricle during ventricular systole. (approximately 100 mm Hg)

The oxygen saturation of blood in the coronary sinus is approximately 60%.

The oxygen saturation of pulmonary vein blood is 98%.

PRINCIPLES of FLOW

Blood flows from a higher pressure chamber to a lower pressure chamber.

The cardiac valves open and close due to a change in pressure.

There will be an increase in the pressure of a chamber located proximal to an obstruction and there will be a decrease in the pressure in the chamber distal to an obstruction. For example, in valvular aortic stenosis the systolic pressure in the proximal chamber, the left ventricle, is increased while pressure in the distal chamber, the aorta, is decreased.

Atrioventricular valve regurgitation will increase the atrial v wave.

Atrioventricular valve stenosis will increase the atrial a wave.

Hypertension and ventricular outflow tract obstruction will increase ventricular systolic pressure.

Congestive heart failure, constrictive pericarditis, restrictive cardiomyopathy and diastolic dysfunction will increase ventricular diastolic pressure.

Left to right shunts, pulmonary hypertension or left heart disease will increase pulmonary artery pressures.

MANEUVERS ALTERING CARDIAC PHYSIOLOGY

Supine to standing, the strain phase of the Valsalva maneuver, inhalation of amyl nitrite and expiration will decrease venous return.

Standing to supine, passive leg raising, standing to squatting and inspiration will increase venous return.

The murmurs of hypertrophic obstructive cardiomyopathy and mitral valve prolapse are increased with a decrease in venous return such as during the strain phase of the Valsalva maneuver, inhalation of amyl nitrite or supine to standing.

The murmurs of hypertrophic obstructive cardiomyopathy and mitral valve prolapse will be decreased with an increase in venous return such as with standing to supine and standing to squatting.

The isometric handgrip increases the murmur of mitral regurgitation, aortic regurgitation and ventricular septal defect and decreases the murmur of aortic stenosis and hypertrophic obstructive cardiomyopathy.

Most right heart sounds and murmurs increase with inspiration and decrease with expiration.

Most left heart sounds and murmurs decrease with inspiration and increase during expiration.

The time interval between the two components of the S2 heart sound, aortic valve closure and pulmonic valve closure, increases during inspiration and decreases with expiration. This is referred to as normal physiologic splitting of the S2 heart sound.

NORMAL HEART SOUND GENERATION and TIMING

S1 is the first normal heart sound and is created by the closure of the atrioventricular valves at the onset of the QRS complex where ventricular pressure exceeds atrial pressure.

S2 is the second normal heart sound and is created by closure of the semilunar valves at the end of the T wave where arterial pressure falls below ventricular pressure.

CARDIOVASCULAR CIRCULATION

The component parts of the circulation includes the aorta, peripheral arteries, arterioles, capillaries, venules and veins.

The three layers of a vessel are the inner layer called the tunica intima, the thick middle layer called the tunica media and the tough outer layer called the tunica adventitia.

The arterioles meter blood to the capillaries.

APPENDIX B

CONTROL MECHANISMS

Cardiac performance depends upon preload, afterload, the inherent property of the heart muscle to contract (contractility), and heart rate.

An increase in preload will enhance cardiac performance to a certain physiologic limit. (Frank-Starling's law of the heart)

An increase in afterload (the resistance the ventricle faces as it ejects blood) generally decreases cardiac performance. (force-velocity relationship)

An important determinant of cardiac performance is myocardial contractility. Myocardial ischemia or infarction decreases cardiac performance.

A decrease in heart rate may improve cardiac performance. (interval-strength relationship)

The autonomic nervous system innervates the heart. The sympathetic nervous system increases excitability, heart rate, conduction speed and contractility. The parasympathetic nervous system decreases excitability, heart rate, conduction speed and contractility.

CORONARY CIRCULATION

Coronary artery blood flow occurs predominantly during ventricular diastole.

A stenosis of 70% or greater is considered to be significant coronary artery disease.

Aortic diastolic blood pressure, left ventricular diastolic pressure, heart rate, collateral coronary circulation and certain metabolic factors all affect coronary circulation.

PROPERTIES of BLOOD: COMPOSITION

Blood has two distinct fractions: formed elements (blood cells) and plasma.

The formed elements of blood are red blood cells (erythrocytes), white blood cells (leukocytes) and platelets (thrombocytes).

Red blood cells make up 45% of the formed elements, white blood cells and platelets approximately 1% each.

Plasma is the fluid the formed elements are suspended and constitutes 55% of blood.

Hematocrit is the percentage of red blood cells present.

Anemia is a decrease in the number of red blood cells.

Polycythemia is an increase in the number of red blood cells.

Leukocytosis is an increase in white blood cells.

Leukopenia is a decrease in white blood cells.

Erythropoesis is the production of red blood cells by the bone marrow.

SYMPTOMS of CARDIAC DISEASES and COMMON CAUSES

Angina pectoris is chest pain related to coronary artery disease.

Cachexia is a state of ill health and is associated with long standing heart disease.

APPENDIX B

Clubbing is the lateral and longitudinal curvature of the nails and is associated with right-to-left cardiac shunts or severe pulmonary disease.

Congestive heart failure is the inability of the heart to meet the metabolic demands of the body. Myocardial dysfunction, pressure overload, volume overload, diastolic dysfunction and increased metabolic demands are all causes of congestive heart failure.

Cor pulmonale is right heart failure due to intrinsic pulmonary disease.

Cyanosis is the bluish discoloration of the skin and mucous membranes and is associated with right-to-left cardiac shunts or severe pulmonary disease.

Dyspnea is shortness of breath and is the main symptom of pulmonary or cardiac disease.

Orthopnea is difficulty breathing while supine and is associated with congestive heart failure.

Paroxysmal nocturnal dyspnea is sudden shortness of breath during sleep and is associated with left heart failure.

Edema is the accumulation of fluid in the cells, tissues and cavities and is associated with heart failure. Pulmonary edema may indicate left heart failure while peripheral edema may indicate right heart failure.

Fever and chills are common presenting symptoms for infective endocarditis.

Hepatomegaly is the enlargement of the liver and is associated with right heart failure.

Hemoptysis is the coughing or spitting up of blood and is associated with mitral stenosis.

Jugular venous distention indicates an increase in right heart pressures.

Nocturia is an increase in the frequency of urination at night and is associated with heart failure.

Palpitations are the uncomfortable awareness of the heart beating and is associated with cardiac arrhythmias, smoking, exercise, stress or the excessive consumption of beverages containing caffeine.

Pectus excavatum/carinatum are thoracic cage abnormalities associated with mitral valve prolapse and Marfan's syndrome.

Syncope is a temporary loss of consciousness and is associated with left ventricular outflow tract obstruction, arrhythmia, angina, myocardial infarction, hypotension and pacemaker failure.

PHYSICAL EXAMINATION and SIGNS

Pulsus alternans is alternating weak and strong heart beats and is associated with severe left ventricular systolic dysfunction.

Pulsus bisfierens is two beats in one and is associated with hypertrophic obstructive cardiomyopathy or severe aortic regurgitation.

Pulsus paradoxus is an exaggeration of the normal decrease in systolic blood pressure with inspiration and is associated with cardiac tamponade.

Pulsus parvus et tardus is a small, weak, late peaking pulse associated with valvular aortic stenosis.

Displacement of the point of maximal impulse (PMI) indicates an enlarged heart.

APPENDIX B

Left parasternal lift is due to the anterior displacement of the right ventricle due to an enlarged left atrium. It is associated with severe, chronic mitral regurgitation.

Left ventricular thrust is the exaggerated amplitude and duration of the normal left ventricular impulse and is associated with left ventricular hypertrophy.

Left ventricular systolic bulge is a larger than normal area of pulsation of the left ventricular apex and is associated with left ventricular aneurysm.

Thrills are palpable manifestations of loud, harsh murmurs and are associated with semilunar valve stenosis as well as ventricular septal defect.

CORRELATION of AUSCULTATORY FINDINGS

There are two normal heart sounds: S1 and S2.

S1 is caused by closure of the atrioventricular valves, mitral valve before tricuspid valve, and may be heard throughout the precordium although it is best heard at the cardiac apex. S1 is the the lub in lub-dup and is a soft, low pitched heart sound.

S2 is caused by the closure of the semilunar valves, aortic before pulmonic, and may be heard throughout the precordium, although it is best heard at the right or left upper sternal border. S2 is the dup in lub-dup and is higher pitched than the first heart sound.

Normally S2 is split upon respiration with the time interval between aortic and pulmonic valve closure increasing with inspiration and decreasing with expiration.

The S3 heart sound is associated with increased early rapid diastolic filling such as in severe valvular regurgitation. An S3 is considered abnormal in patients over the age of 35.

The S4 heart sound is a late diastolic heart sound associated with atrial systole. An S4 indicates a decrease in ventricular compliance such as in acute myocardial infarction or significant semilunar valve stenosis.

A loud S1 is an increase in the intensity of atrioventricular valve closure and is associated with mitral valve/tricuspid valve stenosis.

An opening snap is the sound caused by the sudden halt of the mitral/tricuspid valve opening due to atrioventricular valve stenosis.

An ejection click/sound is an early systolic sound associated with the sudden halting of a stenotic semilunar valve.

Midsystolic click is a high pitched heart sound caused by the sudden tensing of the chordae tendineae in mitral valve prolapse.

Fixed split S2 is the lack of respiratory variation of the aortic and pulmonic valve closure time interval and is associated with atrial septal defect.

Pericardial friction rub is a three component friction sound associated with pericarditis.

Pericardial knock is an early diastolic heart sound associated with constrictive pericarditis.

MURMURS

A murmur is caused by turbulent blood flow moving through the heart and great vessels.

Murmurs are characterized by their location, timing, intensity, configuration, pitch and quality.

The cardiac apex is the mitral area.

The lower left sternal border or xyphoid area is the tricuspid area.

The right upper sternal border is the aortic area.

The left upper sternal border is the pulmonic area.

A grade I murmur is barely audible.

A grade II murmur is faintly heard.

A grade III murmur is moderately loud.

A grade IV murmur is loud.

A grade V murmur is very loud.

A grade VI murmur is loud with a thrill.

The early systolic murmur begins with the first heart sound and ends by midsystole and is associated with a small ventricular septal defect, a large ventricular septal defect with pulmonary hypertension or severe, acute atrioventricular valve regurgitation.

The systolic ejection murmur begins after the semilunar valves open and may be caused by semilunar valve stenosis, aortic/pulmonary artery dilatation or an increase in the rate of ventricular ejection.

Pansystolic (holosystolic) murmurs are present when there is flow between two chambers that have widely different pressures throughout systole. The causes include atrioventricular valve regurgitation, ventricular septal defect or aortopulmonary shunt.

Late systolic murmurs are murmurs that begin well after ejection and indicate the presence of mitral valve prolapse or papillary muscle dysfunction.

Early diastolic murmurs begin immediately after the second heart sound and are caused by semilunar valve regurgitation.

Mid-diastolic and late diastolic murmurs are produced by forward flow across the atrioventricular valves. The causes include atrioventricular valve stenosis, left atrial myxoma, significant mitral regurgitation and large left-to-right shunts.

Continuous murmurs result from blood flow constantly moving from a high pressure area to a low pressure area. The causes of a continuous murmur includes patent ductus arteriosus, systemic arteriovenous fistula, coronary artery originating from the pulmonary artery, or a ruptured sinus of Valsalva aneurysm.

The Valsalva maneuver decreases the intensity of all murmurs except hypertrophic obstructive cardiomyopathy and mitral valve prolapse.

Amyl nitrite will increase forward flow murmurs (i.e. mitral valve stenosis) and left ventricular outflow tract obstruction murmurs. Amyl nitrite will decrease the murmur of aortic regurgitation, mitral regurgitation and ventricular septal defect. Mitral valve prolapse may be enhanced with amyl nitrite inhalation.

Isometric handgrip will increase the intensity of left heart regurgitant murmurs and decrease left heart outflow obstruction murmurs.

ELECTROCARDIOGRAPHY (EKG)

The normal EKG consists of a P wave representing atrial depolarization and contraction, a QRS complex representing ventricular depolarization and contraction and a T wave representing ventricular repolarization.

Normal sinus rhythm is present when the heart rate is regular between 60-100 beats per minute and there is a P wave for every uniform QRS complex.

Sinus bradycardia is present when all complexes are normal but the heart rate is below 60 beats per minute.

Sinus tachycardia is present when all complexes are normal but the heart rate is greater than 100 beats per minute.

Sinus arrhythmia is present when all complexes are normal but the heart rate increases and decreases with respiration.

Sinus pause or arrest is present when the SA node fails to send an impulse for a period of time.

Premature atrial contraction (PAC) is present when normal sinus rhythm is interrupted by an abnormal P wave followed by a QRS complex.

Atrial flutter is the rapid regular fluttering of the atria at a rate of between 250 and 350 times per minute. The P waves are saw toothed in appearance and a QRS complex does not follow each P wave.

Atrial fibrillation is caused by multiple atrial foci with no well defined P waves present. The QRS complex is normal although the ventricular rate is irregular. The atrial rate is between 400 to 700 impulses per minute.

Premature ventricular contraction (PVC) is caused by ectopic foci in the ventricle. The PVC occurs early in the cycle, the QRS complex is wide and bizarre looking, and is followed by a compensatory pause.

Ventricular tachycardia is three or more consecutive PVC's with a heart rate of between 150 to 200 beats per minute.

Ventricular fibrillation (cardiac arrest) is present when the myocardium lacks effective muscular contraction.

First degree atrioventricular (AV) block is present when the PR interval is greater than 0.20 seconds.

Second degree AV block is manifested on the electrocardiogram as some P waves being delivered to the ventricles while others are not. In Mobitz I (Wenckebach) there is progressive lengthening of the PR interval until a beat is blocked. In Mobitz II, some beats are conducted while others are not.

APPENDIX B

Third degree AV block, also referred to as complete heart block, is present when no atrial impulse will activate the ventricles. The P waves and QRS complexes occur independent of each other.

The artificial pacemaker will cause the pacemaker artifact (blip) which demonstrates that an impulse has been sent. The QRS complex may be wider than normal.

A pacemaker spike will appear in front of each QRS complex if the pacemaker is located in the ventricle.

If the pacemaker is located in the atria, a pacemaker spike will appear in front of each P wave.

If the pacemaker is located in the atria and ventricle, a pacemaker spike will appear before each P wave and QRS complex.

EXERCISE and PHARMOCOLOGICAL STRESS TESTING

Exercise stress testing may be used to evaluate the cardiovascular response to exercise.

An increase in myocardial oxygen demand during exercise must be met by an increase in coronary artery blood flow or myocardial ischemia will result.

The indications for an exercise stress test include chest pain, assessment of cardiovascular fitness, evaluation of arrhythmia and evaluation of the asymptomatic patient with risk factors.

The most reliable exercise stress test indicator for the presence of coronary artery disease is ST segment depression.

Dobutamine is a positive inotrope and chronotrope that will increase myocardial oxygen consumption.

Dipyridamole (Persantine) will dilate the coronary arteries and induce myocardial ischemia in myocardium supplied by stenotic coronary arteries.

Adenosine is a potent coronary artery vasodilator which may induce hypoperfusion in myocardium supplied by stenotic coronary arteries.

CARDIAC CATHETERIZATION

Cardiac catheterization is an invasive procedure used to visualize cardiac chambers and the coronary arterial system by introducing a catheter into the heart and great vessels.

A routine cardiac catheterization involves a right heart catheterization, left heart catheterization and a coronary arteriogram.

A right heart catheterization involves the evaluation of the pressures and oxygen saturations of the right atrium, right ventricle, pulmonary artery and pulmonary artery wedge.

A right heart catheterization may include a right ventriculogram which is the injection of a radiopaque dye into the right ventricle. Right ventricular global and segmental function and the severity of tricuspid regurgitation may be evaluated.

A right heart catheterization may include a pulmonary artery arteriogram which is the injection of a radiopaque dye into the pulmonary artery. Pulmonary thrombosis or pulmonary artery stenosis may be evaluated by this technique.

A right heart catheterization may include the evaluation of direct left atrial pressure by puncturing and then crossing the interatrial septum with a catheter. This is referred to as the Brockenbraugh procedure.

A left heart catheterization involves the evaluation of the pressures and oxygen saturations of the left ventricle and aorta.

An aortogram (aortography) may be included in a left heart catheterization and is the injection of a radiopaque dye into the ascending aorta in order to evaluate the severity of aortic regurgitation and the dimension of the ascending aorta.

A left ventriculogram may be included in a left heart catheterization and is the injection of a radiopaque dye into the left ventricle. The evaluation of left ventricular function and the severity of mitral regurgitation may be accomplished by a left ventriculogram.

Coronary arteriography is the evaluation of the coronary arterial system with the injection of a radiopaque dye into the right and left coronary arteries. A decrease in a coronary artery diameter of 70% or greater is considered significant coronary artery disease.

The most common method for determining cardiac output in the cardiac catheterization laboratory is the thermodilution method which involves injecting a chilled saline into the right heart and evaluating the temperature change downstream.

The indicator dilution method for predicting cardiac output requires the injection of a dye into the right heart and monitoring the concentration of dye at an arterial site downstream.

The Fick method is the most accurate method for predicting cardiac output in the cardiac catheterization laboratory and involves the measurement of the differences in oxygen content between the arterial and pulmonary systems.

Angiography may be used to predict cardiac output by providing ventricular systolic and diastolic volumes.

The Gorlin formula is used to determine valve area in the cardiac catheterization laboratory.

Oximetry allows for the evaluation of intracardiac shunts by comparing the oxygen content for each cardiac chamber. An oxygen step-up of 10% or more may indicate the presence of an intracardiac left-to-right shunt.

The cardiac catheterization laboratory may calculate the pressure difference (pressure gradient) between two chambers three ways: peak to peak gradient, mean gradient and peak (maximum) instantaneous gradient.

The peak to peak pressure gradient compares the peak systolic pressure of the ventricles to the peak systolic pressures of the great arteries. Cardiac Doppler cannot predict peak to peak pressure gradients.

The mean pressure gradient measures the pressure gradient between two chambers over time. The cardiac catheterization mean gradient should compare well with the cardiac Doppler mean gradient.

The peak (maximum) instantaneous pressure gradient measures the maximum pressure difference between two cardiac chambers. Cardiac catheterization does not routinely report out this gradient although the cardiac Doppler peak instantaneous gradient should match the cardiac catheterization peak instantaneous gradient when measured by the catheterization laboratory.

The cardiac catheterization mean pressure gradient should correlate closely with the cardiac Doppler mean pressure gradient.

The cardiac Doppler peak instantaneous pressure gradient will usually be greater than the cardiac catheterization peak to peak pressure gradient.

CHEST X-RAY

Cardiomegaly on chest x-ray may suggest the presence of pericardial effusion, dilated cardiomyopathy, or ventricular hypertrophy/dilatation.

Increased pulmonary vascularity on chest x-ray may indicate the presence of left heart failure, a left-to-right shunt or left heart valvular disease.

A widened mediastinum may indicate aortic aneurysm, aortic dissection or tumor.

NUCLEAR CARDIOLOGY

Myocardial perfusion imaging utilizes the radioisotope Thallium-201 to evaluate the presence and severity of coronary artery disease. A cold spot will be displayed in areas with myocardial ischemia or infarction.

Infarct avid imaging uses the radioisotope technetium-99 pyrophosphate to detect myocardial infarction. A hot spot will be displayed in the area of myocardial infarction.

Radionuclide angiography (MUGA) may be used to evaluate right heart and left heart ventricular ejection fraction, valvular regurgitation and intracardiac shunts.

BLOOD FLOW DYNAMICS

The factors that influence the flow of fluids through a tube are the pressure gradient, tube radius, tube length and fluid viscosity. (Poiseuille's law)

As the pressure gradient increases, flow volume increases.

As the tube radius increases, flow volume increases.

As tube length increases, flow volume decreases.

As fluid viscosity increases, flow volume decreases.

The tube's radius exerts the greatest influence on flow volume.

Poiseuille's formula may be rearranged in order to predict the resistance to flow through a tube. An increase in fluid viscosity and/or tube length will increase resistance. A change in the tube's radius exerts the greatest influence and is directly related to flow resistance.

Laminar flow is flow in which the fluid layers slide over each other in a smooth, orderly manner. Laminar flow is considered normal flow.

Inlet (plug) flow occurs at the entrance of great vessels and is flow where the velocities are equal at radical distances from the center of the tube.

Fully developed laminar flow will become parabolic as it travels in a tube.

Disturbed flow occurs at an area of stenosis or vessel bifurcation where the fluid particles still flow in a forward direction but have been disturbed.

APPENDIX B

Inlet, parabolic and disturbed flow are types of laminar flow.

Turbulent flow is present when the fluid particles move in multiple directions and different velocities.

The Reynolds number predicts when turbulent flow will occur. Generally, turbulent flow is considered present if the Reynolds number exceeds 2000.

In cardiovascular applications the velocity of blood flow and the diameter of the vessel or valve determines the presence and degree of turbulent flow.

The Bernoulli equation is an expression of the conservation of energy principle which implies that there will be a drop in pressure (potential) energy with an increase in velocity (kinetic) energy.

The simplified Bernoulli equation is $PG = 4 \times (V_2)^2$, where PG is the pressure gradient between two chambers, V_2 is the velocity at the site of the obstruction.

The simplified Bernoulli equation ignores the velocity proximal to the obstruction, viscous friction and flow acceleration.

The lengthened Bernoulli equation, $4 \times (V_2^{\approx} - V_1^{\approx})$ should be utilized whenever the velocity proximal to an obstruction (V_1) exceeds 1.0 m/s such as may be seen in patients with valvular aortic stenosis or aortic coarctation.

EFFECTS of ABNORMAL PRESSURES and LOADING, VOLUME CONCEPTS

Semilunar valve stenosis is a pressure overload of the ventricles initially causing ventricular hypertrophy followed by ventricular dilatation when ventricular failure occurs.

Atrioventricular stenosis is a pressure overload of the atria with atrial dilatation and a potential for pressure to be reflected backwards.

Semilunar valve regurgitation is a volume overload of the ventricle with ventricular dilatation occurring first followed by ventricular hypertrophy.

Atrioventricular valve regurgitation is a volume overload of the atria with atrial dilatation coupled with ventricular dilatation long term.

Atrial septal defect is a volume overload of the right atrium, right ventricle, main pulmonary artery and pulmonary circulation.

Ventricular septal defect is a volume overload of the pulmonary circulation, left atrium and left ventricle.

Patent ductus arteriosus is a volume overload of the pulmonary circulation, left atrium and left ventricle.

Intrinsic pulmonary disease is a pressure overload of the right ventricle with initial right ventricular hypertrophy followed by right ventricular dilatation. (cor pulmonale)

Cardiac tamponade results in the equalization of diastolic cardiac chamber pressures due to the increase in intrapericardial pressures. This increase in intrapericardial pressure will decrease ventricular diastolic filling, stroke volume and cardiac output.

Constrictive pericarditis is the abnormal thickening of the pericardium resulting in a decrease in ventricular diastolic filling.

APPENDIX B

Hypertrophic obstructive cardiomyopathy is a pressure overload of the left ventricle.

Dilated cardiomyopathy initially results in a volume overload of the ventricles and atria.

Restrictive cardiomyopathy results in an increase in ventricular and atrial diastolic pressures.

APPENDIX B

APPENDIX C
THE CARDIOVASCULAR PRINCIPLES 500

1. The heart is a:
   a. system
   b. pump
   c. series
   d. vessel

2. The heart pumps blood in a:
   a. circle
   b. row
   c. series
   d. system

3. The right atrium receives blood from all of the following except the:
   a. superior vena cava
   b. inferior vena cava
   c. coronary sinus
   d. pulmonary veins

4. The muscle bundles that striate the right atrial free wall and atrial appendage are called:
   a. trabeculae
   b. papillary
   c. chordal
   d. pectinate

5. The inferior vena cava's entrance into the right atrium is guarded by the vestigial valve called the:
   a. thebesian
   b. eustachian
   c. papillary
   d. pectinate

6. The fenestrated portion of the eustachian valve is the:
   a. Chiari network
   b. chordal web
   c. eustachian valve
   d. limbus

APPENDIX C

7. The vestigial valve that guards the opening of the coronary sinus as it enters the right atrium is the:
   a. Chiari
   b. eustachian
   c. limbus
   d. thebesian

8. The left atrium normally receives oxygenated blood from the:
   a. pulmonary artery
   b. pulmonary veins
   c. fossa ovalis
   d. aortic valve

9. The central portion of the interatrial septum in the fetus is called the:
   a. limbus
   b. fossa ovalis
   c. foramen ovale
   d. ductus arteriosus

10. The closed central portion of the interatrial septum in the adult is called the:
    a. limbus
    b. fossa ovalis
    c. foramen ovale
    d. ductus arteriosus

11. In approximately what percentage of the adult population is the foramen ovale probe patent?
    a. 0%
    b. 25%
    c. 50%
    d. 75%

12. All of the following are contained in the ventricles of the heart except the:
    a. trabeculae carneae
    b. papillary muscles
    c. chordae tendineae
    d. pectinate muscles

13. The cardiac chamber located most anterior is the:
    a. right atrium
    b. left atrium
    c. right ventricle
    d. left ventricle

APPENDIX C

14. All of the following are papillary muscles of the right ventricle except the:
    a. anterior
    b. conal
    c. posterior
    d. lateral

15. The subpulmonic area of the right ventricle is called the:
    a. infundibulum
    b. oblique margin
    c. sulcus
    d. inflow tract

16. The muscle bundle that stretches from the free wall of the right ventricle to the interventricular septum is the:
    a. septal band
    b. parietal band
    c. moderator band
    d. papillary muscle

17. The muscle bundle which arches from the anterolateral wall to the septal wall in the right ventricle is the:
    a. moderator band
    b. parietal band
    c. septal band
    d. crista supraventricularis

18. The cardiac chamber with the thickest wall is the:
    a. left atrium
    b. right atrium
    c. left ventricle
    d. right ventricle

19. The cardiac chamber which normally forms the cardiac apex is the:
    a. left atrium
    b. right atrium
    c. left ventricle
    d. right ventricle

20. The two papillary muscle groups of the left ventricle are the:
    a. anterior, medial
    b. anterolateral, posteromedial
    c. inferolateral; posteromedial
    d. lateral, anterior

21. The geometric shape the normal left ventricle most closely resembles is the:
    a. circle
    b. pyramid
    c. ellipse
    d. square

22. The two anatomic components of the interventricular septum are called:
    a. supracristal, trabecular
    b. inlet, outlet
    c. subaortic, subpulmonic
    d. membranous, muscular

23. The interventricular septum normally bows towards which cardiac chamber?
    a. left atrium
    b. right atrium
    c. left ventricle
    d. right ventricle

24. All of the following are considered atrioventricular valves except the:
    a. mitral
    b. bicuspid
    c. tricuspid
    d. aortic

25. All of the following are considered components of the atrioventricular valves except the:
    a. annulus
    b. chordae tendineae
    c. papillary muscle
    d. sinus of Valsalva

26. The right heart atrioventricular valve is the:
    a. mitral
    b. aortic
    c. tricuspid
    d. mitral

27. The names of the tricuspid valve leaflets include all of the following except:
    a. anterior
    b. medial
    c. septal
    d. left

APPENDIX C

28. Blood flow across the atrioventricular valves normally occurs during:
    a. ventricular diastole
    b. isovolumic relaxation
    c. ventricular systole
    d. isovolumic contraction

29. Atrioventricular valve regurgitation occurs during:
    a. ventricular diastole
    b. isovolumic relaxation
    c. ventricular systole
    d. atrial systole

30. The left heart atrioventricular valve is the:
    a. mitral
    b. aortic
    c. pulmonic
    d. tricuspid

31. The mitral valve is located between which two cardiac chambers?
    a. left atrium, right atrium
    b. left atrium, left ventricle
    c. right atrium, right ventricle
    d. right atrium, left ventricle

32. All of the following are considered components of the mitral valve except:
    a. anterior leaflet
    b. posterior leaflet
    c. nodules
    d. commissures

33. The semilunar valves are situated between the ventricles and the:
    a. atria
    b. great arteries
    c. vena cava
    d. sinuses

34. Normally blood flow across the semilunar valves occurs during:
    a. ventricular diastole
    b. atrial systole
    c. ventricular systole
    d. ventricular diastasis

APPENDIX C

35. Blood flow across the semilunar valves is noted during ventricular diastole. This is considered (a):
    a. normal
    b. stenosis
    c. regurgitation
    d. shunt

36. The right heart semilunar valve is the:
    a. mitral
    b. tricuspid
    c. pulmonic
    d. aortic

37. The names of the pulmonic valve cusps include all of the following except:
    a. anterior
    b. medial
    c. posterior
    d. left

38. The left heart semilunar valve is the:
    a. mitral
    b. aortic
    c. pulmonic
    d. tricuspid

39. The names of the aortic valve cusps include all of the following except:
    a. right
    b. left
    c. non
    d. anterior

40. The most common congenital heart defect found in the adult population is (the):
    a. Ebstein's anomaly
    b. coarctation
    c. bicuspid aortic valve
    d. d-transposition of the great arteries

41. The vessel that carries oxygenated blood from the left ventricle to the body is the:
    a. aorta
    b. pulmonary artery
    c. coronary
    d. capillary

APPENDIX C

    b.   aortic isthmus
    c.   ascending aorta
    d.   abdominal aorta

43. The section of the aorta located between the brachiocephalic artery and the left subclavian artery is the:
    a.   aortic annulus
    b.   transverse aorta
    c.   descending thoracic aorta
    d.   abdominal aorta

44. The section of the aorta located between the left subclavian artery and the diaphragm is the:
    a.   ascending aorta
    b.   aortic arch
    c.   descending thoracic aorta
    d.   abdominal aorta

45. The section of the aorta located between the diaphragm and the iliac arteries is the:
    a.   ascending aorta
    b.   transverse aorta
    c.   abdominal aorta
    d.   descending thoracic aorta

46. The section of the aorta that is located between the left subclavian artery and the insertion of the ligamentum arteriosum is the:
    a.   ascending aorta
    b.   aortic arch
    c.   aortic annulus
    d.   aortic isthmus

47. All of the following are vessels that originate from the aortic arch except the:
    a.   left subclavian
    b.   left common carotid artery
    c.   left superior vena cava
    d.   brachiocephalic

48. The coronary arteries originate from the:
    a.   oblique sinus
    b.   sinuses of Valsalva
    c.   transverse sinus
    d.   atrioventricular groove

APPENDIX C

49. In the majority, all of the following receive oxygenated blood from the right coronary artery except:
    a. right atrium
    b. right ventricle
    c. inferior wall of the left ventricle
    d. anterolateral wall of the left ventricle

50. Which of the following coronary artery branches provide oxygenated blood to the inferior wall of the heart?
    a. left anterior descending
    b. posterior descending
    c. oblique marginal
    d. acute margin

51. All of the following are left heart coronary artery branches except:
    a. left anterior descending
    b. left circumflex
    c. acute margin
    d. diagonal

52. Which of the following coronary arteries provides oxygenated blood to the anterior interventricular septum?
    a. left anterior descending
    b. left circumflex
    c. oblique marginal
    d. posterior descending

53. The _____ artery connects the right ventricle to the pulmonary artery branches.
    a. coronary
    b. brachiocephalic
    c. pulmonary
    d. subclavian

54. Which of the following arteries carries deoxygenated blood?
    a. aorta
    b. pulmonary
    c. common carotid
    d. innominate

55. The coronary sinus lies in the:
    a. anterior interventricular sulcus
    b. posterior atrioventricular sulcus
    c. coronary sulcus
    d. posterior descending interventricular sulcus

APPENDIX C

56. Which of the following collects deoxygenated blood from the coronary circulation?
    a.   superior vena cava
    b.   inferior vena cava
    c.   coronary sinus
    d.   left anterior descending

57. All of the following are considered a part of the coronary sinus system except the:
    a.   great cardiac vein
    b.   arterioluminal
    c.   middle cardiac vein
    d.   small cardiac vein

58. The great cardiac vein drains all of the following coronary arteries except the:
    a.   right coronary artery
    b.   left main coronary artery
    c.   left anterior descending
    d.   left circumflex

59. The middle cardiac vein drains the:
    a.   left main coronary artery
    b.   left anterior descending
    c.   left circumflex
    d.   posterior descending artery

60. Which of the following has the lowest oxygen saturation?
    a.   pulmonary veins
    b.   coronary sinus
    c.   superior vena cava
    d.   inferior vena cava

61. The pacemaker of the heart is the:
    a.   sinoatrial node
    b.   internodal tracts
    c.   atrioventricular node
    d.   Purkinje fibers

APPENDIX C

62. The sinoatrial node is located near the entrance of the:
    a. superior vena cava
    b. inferior vena cava
    c. pulmonary veins
    d. coronary sinus

63. The most developed of the internodal pathways which delivers the impulse from the sinoatrial node to the left atrium is called:
    a. Thorel's
    b. Wenckebach's
    c. Bachmann's
    d. Chiari's

64. Which of the following components of the cardiac conduction system delays the impulse 1/10th of a second to allow the atria to deliver blood to the ventricles?
    a. sinoatrial node
    b. internodal pathways
    c. atrioventricular node
    d. His bundle

65. The portion of the cardiac conduction system that electrically connects the atria to the ventricles is called the:
    a. sinoatrial node
    b. atrioventricular node
    c. His bundle
    d. Purkinje fibers

66. Which components of the cardiac conduction system delivers the electrical impulse from the bundle of His to the Purkinje fibers?
    a. sinoatrial node
    b. atrioventricular node
    c. Purjinje fibers
    d. bundle branches

67. Which portion of the electrical conduction system delivers the electrical impulse to the ventricular heart walls?
    a. Purkinje fibers
    b. bundle branches
    c. atrioventricular node
    d. sinoatrial node

APPENDIX C

68. Which of the following is arranged in the sequence that cardiac conduction normally occurs?
   a. SA node - Bundle branches - AV node - Purkinje fibers - Internodal tracts - His bundle
   b. AV node - SA node - Purkinje fibers - Internodal tracts - His bundle - Bundle branches
   c. SA node - Internodal tracts - AV node - His bundle - Bundle branches - Purkinje fibers
   d. Internodal tracts - His bundle - Bundle branches - Purkinje fibers - SA node - AV node

69. Ventricular depolarization occurs from:
   a. endocardium to epicardium
   b. epicardium to endocardium
   c. varies
   d. cannot be predicted

70. The thin outer layer directly adherent to the heart is called the:
   a. epicardium
   b. myocardium
   c. endocardium
   d. parietal

71. The thick, muscular layer of the heart is called the:
   a. epicardium
   b. endocardium
   c. myocardium
   d. fibrous

72. The thin inner layer of the heart is called the:
   a. myocardium
   b. endocardium
   c. epicardium
   d. parietal

73. The cardiac adipose tissue lies between which two layers of the heart?
   a. myocardium and endocardium
   b. epicardium to endocardium
   c. endocardium and myocardium
   d. epicardium and myocardium

74. The heart is placed in a protective sac called the:
   a. visceral pericardium
   b. parietal serous pericardium
   c. parietal pericardium
   d. oblique sinus

75. The pericardial space is located between the:
    a. parietal serous pericardium and epicardium
    b. fibrous pericardium and endocardium
    c. epicardium and myocardium
    d. visceral pericardium and myocardium

76. The pericardial space normally contains up to _____ cc of pericardial fluid.
    a. 0
    b. 50
    c. 100
    d. 200

77. The free space created by the pericardial - pulmonary vein interface behind the left atrium is the:
    a. carotid sinus
    b. oblique sinus
    c. transverse sinus
    d. coronary sinus

78. The free space created by the pericardial - great vessel interface is called the:
    a. carotid sinus
    b. oblique sinus
    c. transverse sinus
    d. coronary sinus

79. The thin moist membrane that lines the fibrous pericardium is the:
    a. visceral pericardium
    b. epicardium
    c. parietal serous
    d. parietal pericardium

80. The tip of the heart formed by the left ventricle is called the:
    a. base
    b. apex
    c. sinus
    d. pericardium

81. The widest portion of the heart is called the:
    a. apex
    b. base
    c. sinus
    d. pericardium

APPENDIX C

82. The junction where the left heart border meets the pleura is called the:
    a. transverse sinus
    b. parietal serous
    c. oblique margin
    d. acute margin

83. Where the right heart border meets the diaphragm is the:
    a. transverse sinus
    b. oblique margin
    c. parietal serous
    d. acute margin

84. In relation to the aorta, the pulmonary artery lies:
    a. anterior and medial
    b. posterior and lateral
    c. anterior and leftward
    d. posterior and rightward

85. Which of the following cardiac valves lies closest to the cardiac apex?
    a. mitral
    b. aortic
    c. tricuspid
    d. pulmonic

86. The heart tube appears by day:
    a. one
    b. ten
    c. twenty one
    d. forty three

87. The heart is completely formed by week:
    a. one
    b. three
    c. seven
    d. ten

88. The heart tube loops:
    a. anterior and rightward
    b. medially and laterally
    c. posterior and leftward
    d. caudad and coronal

APPENDIX C

89. The sinus venosus contributes to the formation of all of the following except the:
    a. superior vena cava
    b. inferior vena cava
    c. coronary sinus
    d. pulmonary veins

90. All of the following are a part of the interatrial septum except the:
    a. bulbus cordis
    b. septum primum
    c. septum secundum
    d. foramen ovale

91. The atrioventricular canal is divided by the:
    a. sinus venosus
    b. septum primum
    c. interventricular septum
    d. endocardial cushions

92. The endocardial cushions contribute to the formation of all of the following except the:
    a. semilunar valves
    b. atrioventricular valves
    c. atrial septum
    d. membranous septum

93. The primitive ventricle is most often a morphologic:
    a. right ventricle
    b. left ventricle
    c. varies
    d. cannot be predicted

94. The bulbus cordis contributes to the formation of all of the following except the:
    a. right ventricle
    b. left ventricle outflow tract
    c. right ventricle outflow tract
    d. ductus arteriosus

95. Which of the following is considered a cono-truncal abnormality?
    a. bicuspid aortic valve
    b. patent ductus arteriosus
    c. tetralogy of Fallot
    d. univentricular heart

APPENDIX C

96. The aortic sac contributes to the formation of all of the following except the:
    a. bulboventricular foramen
    b. internal carotid artery
    c. aortic arch
    d. pulmonary artery branches

97. The exchange of oxygen and carbon dioxide occurs in the maternal:
    a. lungs
    b. placenta
    c. heart
    d. renals

98. Which of the following carries oxygenated blood to the fetus?
    a. umbilical vein
    b. umbilical arteries
    c. maternal placenta
    d. foramen ovale

99. Which of the following connects the umbilical vein to the inferior vena cava?
    a. foramen ovale
    b. truncus arteriosus
    c. umbilical artery
    d. ductus venosus

100. Which of the following permits the flow of blood from the right atrium to the left atrium during fetal circulation?
    a. ductus arteriosus
    b. ductus venosus
    c. umbilical artery
    d. foramen ovale

101. In fetal circulation, which of the following allows blood to be shunted from the pulmonary artery to the aorta?
    a. foramen ovale
    b. ductus arteriosus
    c. ductus venosus
    d. ligamentum arteriosum

102. During fetal circulation, deoxygenated blood is returned to the placenta via the:
    a. foramen ovale
    b. ductus arteriosus
    c. umbilical vein
    d. umbilical arteries

APPENDIX C

103. All of the following are true statements concerning postnatal circulation except:
    a.   pulmonary vascular resistance increases
    b.   foramen ovale closes due to an increase in left heart pressures
    c.   ductus arteriosus closes due to flow of oxygenated blood across the ductus arteriosus
    d.   ductus venosus closes and becomes the ligamentum venosum

104. The atrial septal defect that involves the central portion of the atrial septum is the:
    a.   ostium secundum
    b.   ostium primum
    c.   sinus venosus
    d.   coronary sinus

105. The atrial septal defect that involves the upper portion of the atrial septum is called the:
    a.   coronary sinus
    b.   sinus venosus
    c.   ostium primum
    d.   ostium secundum

106. The atrial septal defect that involves the lower portion of the atrial septum is called the:
    a.   sinus venosus
    b.   ostium primum
    c.   ostium secundum
    d.   patent foramen ovale

107. Which atrial septal defect is associated with mitral valve prolapse?
    a.   ostium primum
    b.   ostium secundum
    c.   sinus venosus
    d.   coronary sinus

108. Which atrial septal defect is associated with partial anomalous pulmonary venous return?
    a.   ostium secundum
    b.   ostium primum
    c.   coronary sinus
    d.   sinus venosus

109. Which atrial septal defect is associated with cleft atrioventricular valve?
    a.   sinus venosus
    b.   coronary sinus
    c.   ostium primum
    d.   ostium secundum

APPENDIX C

a. ostium secundum
b. ostium primum
c. coronary sinus
d. sinus venosus

111. Which atrial septal defect is associated with Lutembacher's syndrome?
    a. ostium primum
    b. sinus venosus
    c. coronary sinus
    d. ostium secundum

112. The ventricular septal defect located beneath the aortic valve at the level of the left ventricular outflow tract is the:
    a. perimembranous
    b. muscular
    c. inlet
    d. outlet

113. The ventricular septal defect which involves the muscular septum and may be multiple is the:
    a. perimembranous
    b. trabecular
    c. inlet
    d. outlet

114. The ventricular septal defect located posteriorly and inferiorly beneath the right heart atrioventricular valve is the:
    a. outlet
    b. trabecular
    c. inlet
    d. perimembranous

115. The ventricular septal defect located beneath the pulmonic valve in the right ventricular outflow tract is the:
    a. outlet
    b. perimembranous
    c. inlet
    d. trabecular

116. The abnormal narrowing of the descending thoracic aorta is called:
    a. truncus
    b. coarctation
    c. Ebstein's
    d. Uhl's anomaly

117. The congenital heart defect most often associated with aortic coarctation is the:
    a. cleft atrioventricular valve
    b. perimembranous ventricular septal defect
    c. ostium secundum atrial septal defect
    d. bicuspid aortic valve

118. All of the following are considered components of tetralogy of Fallot except:
    a. subpulmonic stenosis
    b. malalignment vetricular septal defect
    c. ostium primum atrial septal defect
    d. overriding aorta

119. The aorta arises from the right ventricle and the pulmonary artery arises from the left ventricle. This is called:
    a. normal
    b. d-transposition of the great arteries
    c. Ebstein's anomaly
    d. l-transposition of the great arteries

120. Ventricular inversion with the aorta orginating from the right ventricle and the pulmonary artery originating from the left ventricle is called:
    a. tetralogy of Fallot
    b. Turner's syndrome
    c. d-transposition of the great arteries
    d. l-transposition of the great arteries

121. A single great vessel that gives rise to the pulmonary arteries, coronary arteries and arch vessels is called:
    a. truncus arteriosus
    b. tetralogy of Fallot
    c. l-transposition of the great arteries
    d. d-transposition of the great arteries

122. The failure of the pulmonary vascular resistance to fall after birth thus resulting in right-to left foramen ovale and ductus arteriosus shunts is called:
    a. tetralogy of Fallot
    b. d-transposition of the great arteries
    c. persistent fetal circulation
    d. patent foramen ovale

123. Which of the following is most likely to be associated with paradoxical embolism in the adult?
    a. bicuspid aortic valve
    b. patent foramen ovale
    c. cleft atrioventricular valve
    d. aortic coarctation

APPENDIX C

124. All of the following are associated with persistent ductus arteriosus except:
    a.   prematurity
    b.   maternal rubella
    c.   maternal diabetes
    d.   high altitude birth

125. The abnormal insertion of the tricuspid valve towards the cardiac apex is called:
    a.   Ebstein's anomaly
    b.   Turner's syndrome
    c.   Down's syndrome
    d.   Ehlers-Danlos

126. All of the following are generally considered left-to-right shunts except:
    a.   atrial septal defect
    b.   ventricular septal defect
    c.   persistent fetal circulation
    d.   patent ductus arteriosus

127. The period of time the ventricles are filling with blood is called:
    a.   ventricular systole
    b.   ventricular diastole
    c.   isovolumic contraction
    d.   isovolumic relaxation

128. According to the electrocardiogram, ventricular diastole occurs between the:
    a.   QRS and T wave
    b.   P wave to the QRS complex
    c.   end of the T wave to the onset of the QRS complex
    d.   S wave to the P wave

129. Which of the following statements is correct concerning the cardiac valves during ventricular diastole?
    a.   atrioventricular valves open, semilunar valves open
    b.   atrioventricular valves closed, semilunar valves closed
    c.   atrioventricular valves open, semilunar valves closed
    d.   atrioventricular valves closed, semilunar valves open

130. All of the following are considered components of ventricular diastole except:
    a.   atrial systole
    b.   rapid early filling
    c.   diastasis
    d.   pre-ejection period

APPENDIX C

131. What percentage of filling normally occurs during early, rapid ventricular diastole
     a. 10%
     b. 30%
     c. 50%
     d. 70%

132. What percentage of filling normally occurs with atrial systole?
     a. 10%
     b. 30%
     c. 50%
     d. 70%

133. In relation to the electrocardiogram, ventricular systole occurs during the:
     a. end of the T wave to the onset of the QRS complex
     b. peak of the R wave to the end of the S wave
     c. onset of the Q wave to the end of the T wave
     d. end of the P wave to the onset of QRS complex

134. Which of the following is a true statement concerning the cardiac valves during ventricular systole?
     a. semilunar valves are open, atrioventricular valves are open
     b. semilunar valve are closed, atrioventricular valves are closed
     c. semilunar valves are open, atrioventricular valves are closed
     d. semilunar valves are closed, atrioventricular valve are open

135. The time period between semilunar valve closure and atrioventricular valve opening is called:
     a. ventricular systole
     b. atrial systole
     c. isovolumic contraction
     d. isovolumic relaxation

136. Which of the following is a true statement concerning isovolumic relaxation?
     a. ventricular pressure and volume are decreasing
     b. ventricular pressure and volume are increasing
     c. ventricular pressure is decreasing and ventricular volume is increasing
     d. ventricular pressure is decreasing and ventricular volume is unchanged

137. The amount of blood pumped out of the heart per beat is called:
     a. stroke volume
     b. cardiac output
     c. cardiac index
     d. ejection fraction

APPENDIX C

138. The amount of blood pumped out of the heart per minute is called:
    a. stroke volume
    b. cardiac output
    c. cardiac index
    d. ejection fraction

139. Cardiac output adjusted for body surface area is called:
    a. stroke volume
    b. cardiac output
    c. cardiac index
    d. ejection fraction

140. The percentage of blood pumped out of the heart per beat is called:
    a. stroke volume
    b. cardiac output
    c. cardiac index
    d. ejection fraction

141. The formula for stroke volume is:
    a. end-diastolic volume - end systolic volume
    b. end-diastolic volume - end-systolic volume x heart rate
    c. end-diastolic volume - end-systolic volume x heart rate/body surface area
    d. end-diastolic volume - end-systolic volume/end- diastolic volume x 100

142. The formula for cardiac output is:
    a. end-diastolic volume - end-systolic volume
    b. end-diastolic volume - end-systolic volume x heart rate
    c. end-diastolic volume - end-systolic volume x heart rate/body surface area
    d. end-diastolic volume - end-systolic volume/end- diastolic volume x 100

143. The formula for cardiac index is:
    a. end-diastolic volume - end-systolic volume
    b. end-diastolic volume - end-systolic volume x heart rate
    c. end-diastolic volume - end-systolic volume x heart rate/body surface area
    d. end-diastolic volume - end-systolic volume/end- diastolic volume x 100

144. The formula for ejection fraction is:
    a. end-diastolic volume - end-systolic volume
    b. end-diastolic volume - end-systolic volume x heart rate
    c. end-diastolic volume - end-systolic volume x heart rate/body surface area
    d. end-diastolic volume - end-systolic volume/end-diastolic volume x 100

APPENDIX C

145. The normal range for stroke volume is:
    a.   70 cc to 100 cc
    b.   62% $\pm$12%
    c.   2.4 lpm/m^2 to 4.2 lpm/m^2
    d.   4 lpm to 8 lpm

146. The normal range for cardiac output is:
    a.   2.4 lpm/m^2 to 4.2 lpm/m^2
    b.   70 cc to 100 cc
    c.   62% $\pm$12%
    d.   4 lpm to 8 lpm

147. The normal range for cardiac index is:
    a.   62% $\pm$12%
    b.   70 cc to 100 cc
    c.   4 lpm to 8 lpm
    d.   2.4 lpm/m^2 to 4.2 lpm/m^2

148. The normal range for ejection fraction is:
    a.   4 lpm to 8 lpm
    b.   2.4 lpm/m^2 to 4.2 lpm/m^2
    c.   70 cc to 100 cc
    d.   62% $\pm$ 12%

149. All of the following may be calculated by cardiac Doppler except:
    a.   stroke volume
    b.   cardiac output
    c.   cardiac index
    d.   ejection fraction

150. All of the following are considered a part of the pulmonary circulation except:
    a.   right ventricle
    b.   main pulmonary artery and branches
    c.   pulmonary capillaries
    d.   vena cava

151. All of the following are considered a component of the systemic circulation except:
    a.   left ventricle
    b.   aorta
    c.   cerebral, peripheral and abdominal veins
    d.   pulmonary veins

APPENDIX C

152. When comparing the systemic circulation to the pulmonary circulation all of the following are true except:
    a. higher pressure
    b. higher resistance
    c. higher carbon dioxide content
    d. thicker vessel walls

153. If the left ventricular stroke volume is 90 cc, the right ventricular stroke volume should normally be:
    a. 10% greater
    b. 10% less
    c. equal to
    d. cannot be predicted

154. The central venous pressure is 4 mm Hg. This pressure most likely represents which cardiac chamber pressure?
    a. right atrium
    b. left atrium
    c. left ventricle
    d. pulmonary artery

155. A normal pressure tracing reads 134/76 mm Hg. This most likely represents the pressure in the:
    a. right atrium
    b. left atrium
    c. left ventricle
    d. aorta

156. A normal pressure tracing reads 120/12 mm Hg. This most likely represents the pressure in the:
    a. right atrium
    b. left atrium
    c. left ventricle
    d. aorta

157. A pulmonary wedge pressure tracing reads 14 mm Hg. This represents the pressure in the:
    a. right atrium
    b. left atrium
    c. left ventricle
    d. pulmonary artery

158. A normal pressure tracing reads 22/12 mm Hg. This most likely represents the pressure in the:
    a. right atrium
    b. left atrium
    c. left ventricle
    d. pulmonary artery

APPENDIX C

159. A normal pressure tracing reads 22/4 mm Hg. This most likely represents the pressure in the:
    a. right atrium
    b. right ventricle
    c. pulmonary artery
    d. aorta

160. A normal pressure tracing reads 3 mm Hg. This most likely represents the pressure in the:
    a. right atrium
    b. left atrium
    c. pulmonary artery
    d. aorta

161. Blood flow travels from an area of:
    a. high pressure to low pressure
    b. low pressure to high pressure
    c. varies
    d. cannot be predicted

162. Which of the following causes cardiac valves to open and close?
    a. blood flow
    b. pressure change
    c. valve apparatus
    d. cardiac rotational motion

163. Which pressure will most likely be increased initially in a patient with valvular aortic stenosis?
    a. aorta
    b. left ventricle
    c. right atrium
    d. right ventricle

164. Which pressure will most likely be increased initially in a patient with mitral stenosis?
    a. left atrium
    b. left ventricle
    c. right atrium
    d. right ventricle

165. Which of the following atrial waves will most likely be increased in a patient with significant atrioventricular valve regurgitation?
    a. a wave
    b. y descent
    c. v wave
    d. x descent

166. Which of the following atrial waves will most likely be increased in a patient with atrioventricular valve stenosis?
    a. a wave
    b. y descent
    c. v wave
    d. x descent

167. All of the following will increase ventricular systolic pressure except:
    a. systemic hypertension
    b. pulmonary hypertension
    c. semilunar valve stenosis
    d. atrioventricular valve prolapse

168. All of the following may increase ventricular end-diastolic pressure except:
    a. sinus of Valsalva aneurysm
    b. constrictive pericarditis
    c. congestive heart failure
    d. poor ventricular systolic function

169. All of the following may increase pulmonary artery pressure except:
    a. left-to-right shunts
    b. tricuspid regurgitation
    c. left heart disease
    d. chronic obstructive pulmonary disease

170. All of the following maneuvers will increase venous return except:
    a. supine to standing
    b. standing to supine
    c. passive leg raising
    d. standing to squatting

171. Which of the following maneuvers will reduce venous return?
    a. standing to squatting
    b. passive leg raising
    c. standing to supine
    d. supine to standing

172. How will the strain phase of the Valsalva maneuver affect venous return?
    a. increase
    b. decrease
    c. varies
    d. cannot be predicted

173. All of the following will increase during the isometric handgrip except:
    a. peripheral vascular resistance
    b. blood pressure
    c. heart rate
    d. respiratory rate

174. How will quiet inspiration affect venous return?
    a. increase
    b. decrease
    c. varies
    d. cannot be predicted

175. How will quiet expiration affect venous return?
    a. increase
    b. decrease
    c. varies
    d. cannot be predicted

176. All of the following murmurs will decrease in intensity during the maneuver supine to standing except:
    a. semilunar valve stenosis
    b. hypertrophic cardiomyopathy
    c. semilunar valve regurgitation
    d. atrioventricular valve regurgitation

177. Which of the following murmurs will decrease in intensity during the maneuver standing to supine?
    a. valvular aortic stenosis
    b. valvular pulmonic stenosis
    c. hypertrophic cardiomyopathy
    d. cannot be predicted

178. How will the maneuver standing to squatting affect the murmur of hypertrophic cardiomyopathy?
    a. increase
    b. decrease
    c. varies
    d. cannot be predicted

179. All of the following murmurs will decrease in intensity during the strain phase of the Valsalva maneuver except:
    a. valvular aortic stenosis
    b. tricuspid regurgitation
    c. hypertrophic cardiomyopathy
    d. mitral valve stenosis

APPENDIX C

180. Quiet inspiration will increase all of the following except:
    a. tricuspid regurgitation
    b. mitral regurgitation
    c. S2 time interval
    d. pulmonary regurgitation

181. All of the following will decrease during quiet expiration except:
    a. tricuspid regurgitation
    b. pulmonary regurgitation
    c. S2 time interval
    d. mitral regurgitation

182. The normal S1 heart sound is caused by:
    a. atrioventricular valve opening
    b. atrioventricular valve closure
    c. semilunar valve opening
    d. semilunar valve closure

183. In relation to the electrocardiogram, the S1 heart sound normally occurs at the:
    a. onset of the P wave
    b. onset of the QRS
    c. end of the T wave
    d. end of the S wave

184. Normally the loudest component of the S1 heart sound is closure of the:
    a. mitral valve
    b. tricuspid valve
    c. aortic valve
    d. pulmonic valve

185. In relationship to tricuspid valve closure, normally mitral valve closure occurs:
    a. before
    b. during
    c. after
    d. varies

186. The normal S2 heart sound is caused by:
    a. atrioventricular valve closure
    b. atrioventricular valve opening
    c. semilunar valve closure
    d. semilunar valve opening

APPENDIX C

187. In relation to the electrocardiogram, S2 normally occurs at the:
    a. onset of the P wave
    b. onset of the QRS complex
    c. end of the T wave
    d. end of the PR interval

188. Which component of S2 is normally the loudest?
    a. mitral valve opening
    b. tricuspid valve closure
    c. aortic valve closure
    d. pulmonic valve closure

189. Compared to the pulmonic valve, aortic valve closure normally occurs:
    a. before
    b. during
    c. after
    d. varies

190. Which of the following will increase the interval between aortic valve closure and pulmonic valve closure?
    a. inspiration
    b. expiration
    c. standing to supine
    d. strain phase of the Valsalva

191. All of the following are considered vessel wall layers except the:
    a. intima
    b. media
    c. adventia
    d. vasa vasorum

192. Which of the following component parts of the circulation is best capable of altering blood flow to the capillaries?
    a. aorta
    b. peripheral arteries
    c. arterioles
    d. venules

193. Which of the following components of the circulation conducts blood from the peripheral tissues to the heart?
    a. aorta
    b. venules
    c. arterioles
    d. veins

APPENDIX C

194. Which effect will an increase in preload normally have on cardiac contractility?
    a. increase
    b. decrease
    c. varies
    d. cannot be predicted

195. Which of the following will most likely increase ventricular afterload?
    a. atrioventricular valve regurgitation
    b. atrioventricular valve stenosis
    c. semilunar valve regurgitation
    d. semilunar valve stenosis

196. Coronary artery blood occurs predominantly during:
    a. atrial systole
    b. ventricular diastole
    c. ventricular systole
    d. isovolumic contraction

197. Which percent stenosis is considered significant coronary artery disease?
    a. 10%
    b. 30%
    c. 50%
    d. 70%

198. All of the following will affect coronary artery blood flow except:
    a. aortic diastolic blood pressure
    b. left ventricular end-diastolic pressure
    c. heart rate
    d. body surface area

199. All of the following are considered the formed elements of blood except:
    a. plasma
    b. red blod cells
    c. white blood cells
    d. platelets

200. Another term for red blood cells is:
    a. erythrocytes
    b. leukocytes
    c. thrombocytes
    d. plasma

APPENDIX C

201. Another term for white blood cells is:
    a. plasma
    b. thrombocytes
    c. leukocytes
    d. erythrocytes

202. Another term for platelets is:
    a. leukocytes
    b. thrombocytes
    c. erythrocytes
    d. plasma

203. Which component of blood carries hemoglobin?
    a. erythrocytes
    b. leukocytes
    c. plasma
    d. thrombocytes

204. The term that refers to the percentage of red blood cells present is:
    a. leukopenia
    b. anemia
    c. polycthemia
    d. hematocrit

205. The term that means there is an abnormal increase in the number of red blood cells is:
    a. hematocrit
    b. polycythemia
    c. anemia
    d. leukopenia

206. The term used to decribe an abnormal decrease in the number of red blood cells is:
    a. anemia
    b. leukopenia
    c. polycythemia
    d. hematocrit

207. The term that decribes an abnormal increase in the number of white blood cells is:
    a. polycythemia
    b. leukopenia
    c. hematocrit
    d. plasmacrit

APPENDIX C

208. Which of the following terms infers an abnormal decrease in the number of white blood cells?
    a. plasmacrit
    b. hematocrit
    c. leukocytosis
    d. polycythemia

209. What percentage of blood is made up of plasma?
    a. 15%
    b. 35%
    c. 55%
    d. 75%

210. What percentage does red blood cells constitute the formed elements of blood?
    a. 15%
    b. 35%
    c. 55%
    d. 75%

211. Chest pain due to myocardial ischemia is called:
    a. nocturia
    b. clubbing
    c. hemoptysis
    d. angina pectoris

212 _____ is a state of ill health, malnutrition and wasting.
    a. angina pectoris
    b. cachexia
    c. clubbing
    d. edema

213. Which of the following is most likely to be associated with cyanotic congenital heart disease?
    a. cachexia
    b. cor pulmonale
    c. angina pectoris
    d. clubbing

214. The heart's inability to meet the metabolic demands of the body is called:
    a. edema
    b. angina pectoris
    c. congestive heart failure
    d. syncope

215. Right heart failure due to intrinsic pulmonary disease is called:
    a. clubbing
    b. cyanosis
    c. cor pulmonale
    d. angina pectoris

216. The bluish discoloration of the skin and mucous membranes is called:
    a. clubbing
    b. cyanosis
    c. cachexia
    d. cor pulmonale

217. The abnormal uncomfortable awareness of breathing is called:
    a. hemoptysis
    b. hepatomegaly
    c. edema
    d. dyspnea

218. The accumulation of fluid in cells, tissues or cavities is called:
    a. edema
    b. syncope
    c. hemoptysis
    d. nocturia

219. A patient with fever of unknown origin, chills and a new murmur most likely has:
    a. valvular aortic stenosis
    b. mitral valve prolapse
    c. infective endocarditis
    d. cardiac myxoma

220. Which of the following most likely represents right heart failure?
    a. hemoptysis
    b. syncope
    c. hepatomegaly
    d. angina pectoris

221. Which of the following is most often associated with mitral valve stenosis?
    a. cor pulmonale
    b. angina pectoris
    c. hemoptysis
    d. nocturia

APPENDIX C

222. Which of the following indicates increased right heart pressures?
    a. jugular venous distention
    b. hemoptysis
    c. syncope
    d. angina pectoris

223. Excessive urination at night is called:
    a. nocturia
    b. edema
    c. hepatomegaly
    d. cachexia

224. Which of the following is most likely to be associated with mitral valve prolapse?
    a. cachexia
    b. clubbing
    c. pectus excavatum
    d. angina pectoris

225. Which of the following is most likely to be associated with valvular aortic stenosis?
    a. hemoptysis
    b. syncope
    c. pectus carinatum
    d. nocturia

226. Which of the following pulses is most likely to be present in a patient with severe left ventricular dysfunction?
    a. pulsus alternans
    b. pulsus bisfierens
    c. pulsus paradoxus
    d. pulsus parvus et tardus

227. Which of the following pulses is most likely to be present in a patient with hypertrophic cardiomyopathy?
    a. pulsus parvus et tardus
    b. pulsus paradoxus
    c. pulsus bisfierens
    d. pulsus alternans

228. Which of the following pulses is most likely to be present in a patient with cardiac tamponade?
    a. pulsus bisfierens
    b. pulsus alternans
    c. pulsus paradoxus
    d. pulsus parvus et tardus

APPENDIX C

229. Which of the following pulses is most likely to be present in a patient with valvular aortic stenosis?
    a.   pulsus paradoxus
    b.   pulsus bisfierens
    c.   pulsus parvus et tardus
    d.   pulsus alternans

230. Which of the following signs is associated with an enlarged heart?
    a.   thrill
    b.   pectus excavatum
    c.   displacement of the PMI
    d.   left ventricular thrust

231. Which of the following is associated with an enlarged left atrium?
    a.   left parasternal lift
    b.   left ventricular thrust
    c.   left ventricular systolic bulge
    d.   thrill

232. Which of the following signs indicates left ventricular hypertrophy?
    a.   left parasternal lift
    b.   left ventricular thrust
    c.   left ventricular systolic bulge
    d.   thrill

233. Which of the following signs is associated with left ventricular aneurysm?
    a.   left ventricular thrust
    b.   left ventricular systolic bulge
    c.   thrill
    d.   left parasternal lift

234. A palpable murmur is called a:
    a.   left parasternal lift
    b.   left ventricular systolic bulge
    c.   thrill
    d.   left ventricular thrust

235. The first heart sound is caused by:
    a.   closure of the atrioventricular valves
    b.   closure of the semilunar valves
    c.   opening of the atrioventricular valves
    d.   opening of the semilunar valves

APPENDIX C

236. S1 is best auscultated at the:
    a.   right upper sternal border
    b.   left upper sternal border
    c.   xyphoid area
    d.   cardiac apex

237. The second heart sound is caused by the:
    a.   closure of the atrioventricular valves
    b.   closure of the semilunar valves
    c.   opening of the atrioventricular valves
    d.   opening of the semilunar valves

238. S2 is best auscultated at the:
    a.   upper left sternal border
    b.   lower left sternal border
    c.   xyphoid area
    d.   cardiac apex

239. Which of the following are true statements concerning the effect of respiration on S2?
    a.   S2 splits on inspiration; narrows on expiration
    b.   S2 narrows on inspiration, splits on expiration
    c.   S2 reverses on inspiration, normalizes on expiration
    d.   cannot be predicted

240. Which heart sound indicates an increase in early ventricular diastolic filling?
    a.   S1
    b.   S2
    c.   S3
    d.   S4

241. All of the following pathologies are associated with an S3 except:
    a.   mitral stenosis
    b.   anemia
    c.   significant mitral regurgitation
    d.   significant pulmonary regurgitation

242. The S3 is best auscultated at the:
    a.   right upper sternal border
    b.   left upper sternal border
    c.   xyphoid area
    d.   cardiac apex

APPENDIX C

243. Which of the following heart sounds is associated with decreased ventricular compliance?
    a. S1
    b. S2
    c. S3
    d. S4

244. The S4 heart sound occurs in response to:
    a. early ventricular relaxation
    b. isovolumic contraction
    c. atrial systole
    d. ventricular diastasis

245. The S4 heart sound is best auscultated at the:
    a. right upper sternal border
    b. left upper sternal border
    c. xyphoid area
    d. cardiac apex

246. All of the following pathologies are associated with an S4 except:
    a. systemic hypertension
    b. acute myocardial infarction
    c. semilunar valve stenosis
    d. left to right shunt

247. All of the following heart sounds are associated with rheumatic mitral stenosis except:
    a. loud S1
    b. fixed split S2
    c. opening snap
    d. presystolic diastolic rumble

248. Which of the following heart sounds is associated with congenital semilunar valve stenosis?
    a. loud S2
    b. fixed split S2
    c. ejection click
    d. opening snap

249. Which of the following heart sounds is most commonly associated with mitral valve prolapse?
    a. loud S1
    b. opening snap
    c. midsystolic click
    d. fixed split S2

APPENDIX C

250. Which of the following heart sounds is most often associated with atrial septal defect?
    a.   loud S1
    b.   fixed split S2
    c.   midsystolic click
    d.   ejection sound

251. All of the following may cause a murmur except:
    a.   increased flow rate across a cardiac valve
    b.   forward flow across a stenotic valve
    c.   backward flow across a regurgitant valve
    d.   cardiac valve opening and closure

252. For cardiac auscultation, the mitral valve area is considered to be the:
    a.   right upper sternal border
    b.   left upper sternal border
    c.   xyphoid area
    d.   cardiac apex

253. For cardiac auscultation, the tricuspid valve area is considered to be the:
    a.   right upper sternal border
    b.   left upper sternal border
    c.   xyphoid area
    d.   cardiac apex

254. For cardiac auscultation, the aortic valve area is considered to be the:
    a.   right upper sternal border
    b.   left upper sternal border
    c.   xyphoid area
    d.   cardiac apex

255. For cardiac auscultation, the pulmonic valve area is considered to be the:
    a.   right upper sternal border
    b.   left upper sternal border
    c.   xyphoid area
    d.   cardiac apex

256. The description of the timing of a cardiac murmur may include all of the following except:
    a.   diastolic
    b.   diastasis
    c.   systolic
    d.   continuous

APPENDIX C

257. Which grade murmur would be a murmur that is barely heard?
   a.   I
   b.   II
   c.   III
   d.   IV

258. Which grade murmur is described as faintly heard?
   a.   I
   b.   II
   c.   III
   d.   IV

259. Which grade murmur is described as moderately loud?
   a.   I
   b.   II
   c.   III
   d.   IV

260. Which grade murmur is described as loud?
   a.   I
   b.   II
   c.   III
   d.   IV

261. Which grade murmur is described as very loud?
   a.   III
   b.   IV
   c.   V
   d.   VI

262. The grade murmur that may be heard with the stethescope lifted slightly off the chest is:
   a.   III
   b.   IV
   c.   V
   d.   VI

263. A murmur that begins softly and becomes louder is called:
   a.   crescendo
   b.   decrescendo
   c.   crescendo-decrescendo
   d.   diamond shaped

APPENDIX C

264. A murmur that begins loud and becomes softer is called:
    a. crescendo
    b. decrescendo
    c. crescendo-decrescendo
    d. diamond shaped

265. A murmur that begins softly, becomes louder, and then decreases in intensity is called:
    a. crescendo
    b. decrescendo
    c. crescendo-decrescendo
    d. continuous

266. All of the following are associated with an early systolic murmur except:
    a. small ventricular septal defect
    b. valvular aortic stenosis
    c. large ventricular septal defect with pulmonary hypertension
    d. severe acute atrioventricular regurgitation

267. All of the following are associated with a systolic ejection murmur except:
    a. valvular semilunar valve stenosis
    b. dilatation of the aorta or pulmonary artery
    c. increased heart rate
    d. atrioventricular valve regurgitation

268. All of the following are associated with a holosystolic murmur except:
    a. mitral valve regurgitation
    b. semilunar valve stenosis
    c. ventricular septal defect
    d. tricuspid valve regurgitation

269. The most likely cause of a late systolic murmur is:
    a. semilunar valve stenosis
    b. atrioventricular valve stenosis
    c. mitral valve prolapse
    d. patent ductus arteriosus

270. The most likely cause of an early diastolic murmur is:
    a. atrioventricular valve stenosis
    b. atrioventricular valve regurgitation
    c. semilunar valve stenosis
    d. semilunar valve regurgitation

APPENDIX C

271. The most likely cause of a mid-diastolic murmur is:
    a. atrioventricular valve stenosis
    b. mitral valve prolapse
    c. semilunar valve stenosis
    d. semilunar valve regurgitation

272. All of the following are likely causes of a continuous murmur except:
    a. patent ductus arteriosus
    b. atrioventricular valve stenosis
    c. coronary artery from the pulmonary artery
    d. ruptured sinus of Valsalva aneurysm

273. All of the following murmurs will decrease in intensity during the strain phase of the Valsalva maneuver except:
    a. atrioventricular valve stenosis
    b. atrioventricular valve regurgitation
    c. semilunar valve stenosis
    d. hypertrophic cardiomyopathy

274. All of the following are considered a component of a routine cardiac catheterization except:
    a. right heart
    b. left heart
    c. coronary arteriogram
    d. transvalvular Doppler

275. All of the following information may be recorded during a routine cardiac catheterization except:
    a. intracardiac pressures
    b. oxygen saturations
    c. assessment of ventricular function
    d. transvalvular peak velocities

276. All of the following information may be recorded during a routine cardiac catheterization except the evaluation of:
    a. valvular velocities
    b. valvular stenosis/regurgitation
    c. cardiac shunts
    d. congenital heart disease

277. All of the following information may be recorded during a right heart catheterization except:
    a. right atrial pressure
    b. right ventricular systolic/diastolic pressure
    c. left ventricular systolic/diastolic pressure
    d. systolic/mean/diastolic pulmonary artery pressure

APPENDIX C

278. The pulmonary artery wedge pressure is obtained during a:
    a. right heart catheterization
    b. left heart catheterization
    c. coronary arteriogram
    d. pulmonary arteriogram

279. The pulmonary artery wedge pressure represents the pressure of the:
    a. left atrium
    b. right atrium
    c. right ventricle
    d. pulmonary artery

280. Which of the following is the most common right heart cardiac catheterization method used for predicting cardiac output?
    a. Fick
    b. Gorlin
    c. thermodilution
    d. indicator dye

281. All of the following pressures may be obtained during a left heart cardiac catheterization except:
    a. left ventricular systolic
    b. left ventricular end-diastolic
    c. pulmonary wedge pressure
    d. aortic systolic/diastolic

282. Which of the following cardiac catheterization techniques would be best used to evaluate the severity of aortic regurgitation?
    a. aortography
    b. left ventriculography
    c. coronary arteriography
    d. pulmonary wedge

283. All of the following may be evaluated during a cardiac catheterization left ventriculogram except:
    a. mitral regurgitation
    b. left ventricular global function
    c. left ventricular segmental function
    d. left ventricular systolic/end-diastolic pressure

284. The brachial approach that may be utilized during a cardiac catheterization is called the:
    a. Sone's
    b. Judkin's
    c. Gorlin
    d. Fick

APPENDIX C

285. A coronary arteriogram reveals a 75% stenosis of the right coronary artery. This is considered:
    a. normal
    b. mild
    c. moderate
    d. significant

286. The cardiac catheterization technique that injects chilled saline into the right heart and measures the temperature change at a distal site to predict cardiac output is (the):
    a. thermodilution
    b. indicator dilution
    c. Fick method
    d. angiography

287. The cardiac catheterization technique which injects a dye into the right heart and measures the concentration of dye at an arterial site in order to predict cardiac output is called:
    a. thermodilution
    b. indicator dilution
    c. Fick method
    d. angiography

288. The most accurate cardiac catheterization technique for predicting cardiac output is:
    a. thermodilution
    b. indicator dilution
    c. Fick
    d. angiography

289. Which of the following cardiac catheterization techniques allows for the prediction of cardiac output by injecting a radiopaque dye into the ventricle?
    a. Fick
    b. thermodilution
    c. angiography
    d. indicator dilution

290. Which of the following formulas is most often used in the cardiac catheterization laboratory to predict cardiac valve area?
    a. Bernoulli
    b. Bernheim
    c. Gorlin
    d. Fick

291. Which of the following cardiac catheterization techniques would be best to utilize in quantifying a left-to-right shunt?
    a. left ventriculography
    b. aortography
    c. oximetry
    d. arteriography

APPENDIX C

292. The following oxygen saturations were obtained during a right heart catheterization: vena cava: 73%; right atrium: 85%; right ventricle: 85%; and main pulmonary artery: 85%. The most likely diagnosis is:
   a. normal
   b. atrial septal defect
   c. ventricular septal defect
   d. patent ductus arteriosus

293. The following oxygen saturations were obtained during a right heart cardiac catheterization: vena cava: 75%; right atrium: 75%; right ventricle: 75%; and main pulmonary artery: 88%. The most likely diagnosis is:
   a. normal
   b. atrial septal defect
   c. ventricular septal defect
   d. patent ductus arteriosus

294. The following oxygen saturations were obtained during a right heart cardiac catheterization: vena cava: 72%; right atrium: 72%; right ventricle: 84% and main pulmonary artery: 84%. The most likely diagnosis is:
   a. normal
   b. atrial septal defect
   c. ventricular septal defect
   d. patent ductus arteriosus

295. During a cardiac catheterization the forward stroke volume was determined to be 80 cc. The total stroke volume was determined to be 130 cc. The regurgitant volume is:
   a. 0 cc
   b. 50 cc
   c. 130 cc
   d. 210 cc

296. During a cardiac catheterization the total stroke volume was determined to be 100 cc. The forward stroke volume was determined to be 70 cc. The regurgitant fraction is:
   a. 0%
   b. 30%
   c. 70%
   d. 100%

297. The pressure difference between two chambers is called a:
   a. stenosis
   b. gradient
   c. pressure
   d. mean

APPENDIX C

298. The cardiac catheterization technique that compares the peak systolic pressure of the right or left ventricles to the peak systolic pressure of the pulmonary artery or aorta is called:
    a. maximum peak pressure gradient
    b. peak instantaneous gradient
    c. peak-to-peak pressure gradient
    d. mean transvalvular pressure gradient

299. Which cardiac catheterization gradient measures the pressure difference over time?
    a. maximum peak
    b. peak instantaneous
    c. peak-to-peak
    d. mean transvalvular

300. The pressure gradient that reflects the peak pressure difference between two chambers is called:
    a. maximum peak
    b. mean transvalvular
    c. peak-to-peak
    d. peak-to-mean

301. Which of the following cardiac catheterization pressure gradients will best match the cardiac Doppler pressure gradient?
    a. peak instantaneous
    b. maximum instantaeous
    c. peak-to-peak
    d. mean transvalvular

302. A cardiac Doppler examination of a stenotic aortic valve records a peak pressure gradient of 77 mm Hg. The cardiac catheterization peak-to-peak pressure gradient when compared to the cardiac Doppler gradient will most likely be:
    a. equal to
    b. higher
    c. lower
    d. cannot be predicted

303. The cardiac catheterization technique which utilizes the injection of a radiopaque dye into cardiac chambers/great vessels and is recorded on cine film is called:
    a. indicator dilution
    b. angiography
    c. oximetry
    d. thermodilution

APPENDIX C

304. A left ventriculogram will allow the evaluation of all of the following except left ventricular:
    a. global function
    b. segmental function
    c. stroke volume
    d. systolic pressure

305. Which cardiac valve regurgitation may a left ventriculogram best evaluate?
    a. aortic
    b. mitral
    c. pulmonic
    d. tricuspid

306. All of the following may be evaluated during a right heart ventriculogram except right ventricular:
    a. global systolic function
    b. segmental wall motion
    c. tricuspid regurgitation
    d. systolic/diastolic pressure

307. Which cardiac catheterization technique is best used to evaluate aortic root dimension?
    a. coronary arteriogram
    b. left ventriculogram
    c. aortogram
    d. oximetry

308. All of the following are likely causes of cardiomegaly as seen on chest x-ray except:
    a. pleural effusion
    b. dilated cardiomyopathy
    c. ventricular hypertrophy
    d. ventricular dilatation

309. All of the following are associated with an increase in pulmonary vascularity on chest x-ray except:
    a. left heart failure
    b. aortic aneurysm
    c. left-to-right cardiac shunt
    d. left heart valvular disease

310. A widened mediastinum as viewed on a chest x-ray suggests:
    a. infective endocarditis
    b. mitral valve prolapse
    c. aortic dissection
    d. constrictive pericarditis

APPENDIX C

311. Which of the following nuclear medicine tests utilizes Thallium-201 to evaluate coronary artery disease?
    a. myocardial perfusion
    b. infarct avid imaging
    c. radionuclide angiography
    d. MUGA

312. Which of the following nuclear medicine tests is utilized to evaluate acute myocardial infarction?
    a. myocardial perfusion
    b. infarct avid imaging
    c. radionuclide angiography
    d. MUGA

313. Which of the following nuclear medicine tests injects a radionuclide isotope in order to visualize the atria, ventricles and great vessels?
    a. myocardial perfusion
    b. radionuclide angiography
    c. infarct avid imaging
    d. sestamibi imaging

314. Which nuclear medicine test allows for the calculation of ejection fraction?
    a. myocardial perfusion
    b. Cardiolyte
    c. infarct avid imaging
    d. MUGA

315. According to Poiseuille's law, as the pressure gradient increases, flow rate will:
    a. increase
    b. decrease
    c. varies
    d. cannot be predicted

316. According to Poiseuille's law, as the diameter of a tube increases, flow rate will:
    a. increase
    b. decrease
    c. vary
    d. cannot be predicted

317. According to Poiseuille's law, as the length of a tube increases, flow rate:
    a. increases
    b. decreases
    c. varies
    d. cannot be predicted

APPENDIX C

318. According to Poiseuille's law, as fluid viscosity increases, flow rate:
    a.   increases
    b.   decreases
    c.   vary
    d.   cannot be predicted

319. According to Poiseuille's law, which of the following has the greatest effect on flow through a tube?
    a.   pressure gradient
    b.   tube diameter
    c.   tube length
    d.   fluid viscosity

320. Flow in which fluid layers slide over each other in a smooth, orderly manner is called:
    a.   laminar
    b.   disturbed
    c.   turbulent
    d.   outlet

321. Fully developed laminar flow becomes:
    a.   parabolic
    b.   disturbed
    c.   turbulent
    d.   increased

322. Disturbed flow occurs usually at a(n):
    a.   inlet
    b.   bifurcation
    c.   outlet
    d.   annulus

323. _____ flow is present when fluid particles move in multiple directions and different velocities.
    a.   inlet
    b.   laminar
    c.   disturbed
    d.   turbulent

324. The _____ number predicts the onset of turbulent flow.
    a.   Gorlin
    b.   Doppler
    c.   Reynolds
    d.   Bernoulli

325. Which equation allows for the prediction of pressure gradients?
    a. Gorlin
    b. Fick
    c. Bernoulli
    d. Carvallo

326. The velocity across a regurgitant tricuspid valve is 300 cm/s. The predicted pressure gradient would be:
    a. 3 mm Hg
    b. 36 mm Hg
    c. 300 mm Hg
    d. 360,000 mm Hg

327. The clinical use of the simplified Bernoulli equation usually ignores all of the following except:
    a. V_1
    b. V_2
    c. flow acceleration
    d. viscous friction

328. The simplified Bernoulli equation of $4 \times (V_2)^2$ may not be accurate in all of the following situations except:
    a. V_1 velocity greater than 1.0 m/s
    b. tunnel stenosis
    c. discrete stenosis
    d. stenosis in series

329. All of the following are possible causes for congestive heart failure except:
    a. myocardial dysfunction
    b. pressure overload
    c. volume overload
    d. pleural effusion

330. All of the following are possible etiologies for congestive heart failure except:
    a. myocardial ischemia
    b. amyloidosis
    c. aortic aneurysm
    d. valvular aortic stenosis

331. Semilunar valve stenosis is a ventricular:
    a. pressure overload
    b. volume overload
    c. varies
    d. cannot be predicted

APPENDIX C

332. Which effect does semilunar valve stenosis initially have on the ventricle?
   a.   dilatation
   b.   hypertrophy
   c.   varies
   d.   cannot be predicted

333. Atrioventricular valve stenosis is initially a(n):
   a.   atrial volume overload
   b.   atrial pressure overload
   c.   ventricular volume overload
   d.   ventricular pressure overload

334. Which effect does atrioventricular valve stenosis initially have on the atria?
   a.   dilatation
   b.   hypertrophy
   c.   varies
   d.   cannot be predicted

335. Significant chronic semilunar valve regurgitation is initially a ventricular:
   a.   volume overload
   b.   pressure overload
   c.   varies
   d.   cannot be predicted

336. Significant severe acute semilunar valve regurgitation initially causes an increase in:
   a.   ventricular diastolic pressure
   b.   hypertrophy
   c.   varies
   d.   cannot be predicted

337. Significant chronic atrioventricular valve regurgitation initially is a:
   a.   volume overload
   b.   pressure overload
   c.   varies
   d.   cannot be predicted

338. Acute mitral valve regurgitation initially results in:
   a.   atrial/ventricular dilatation
   b.   atrial/ventricular hypertrophy
   c.   pulmonary edema
   d.   cannot be predicted

339. An atrial septal defect initially results in a volume overload of all of the following except:
    a. right atrium
    b. left atrium
    c. right ventricle
    d. pulmonary veins

340. A ventricular septal defect initially results in a volume overload of all of the following except:
    a. right ventricle
    b. left atrium
    c. left ventricle
    d. main pulmonary artery

341. A patent ductus arteriosus initially results in a volume overload of all of the following except:
    a. right ventricle
    b. left atrium
    c. left ventricle
    d. pulmonary veins

342. Intrinsic pulmonary disease results initially in a:
    a. right atrial volume overload
    b. left atrial volume overload
    c. right ventricular pressure overload
    d. left ventricular volume overload

343. Hypertrophic cardiomyopathy is initially a left ventricular:
    a. volume overload
    b. pressure overload
    c. volume/pressure overload
    d. cannot be predicted

344. Dilated cardiomyopathy initially results in a(n):
    a. atrial/ventricular volume overload
    b. atrial/ventricular pressure overload
    c. varies
    d. cannot be predicted

345. A restrictive cardiomyopathy initially results in an increase in atrial and ventricular:
    a. systolic pressure
    b. diastolic pressure
    c. varies
    d. cannot be predicted

APPENDIX C

346. An interatrial septal aneursym usually affects which portion of the interatrial septum?
   a. sinus venosus
   b. foramen ovale
   c. ostium primum
   d. coronary sinus

347. The groove between the right atrium and right ventricle is called the:
   a. coronary sinus
   b. coronary sulcus
   c. crista terminalis
   d. supraventricular crest

348. The left atrium and left ventricle are anteriorly and posteriorly separated by the:
   a. pulmonary veins
   b. coronary artery
   c. atrioventricular groove
   d. posterior descending artery

349. Where all four cardiac chambers meet posteriorly is called the cardiac:
   a. sulcus
   b. sinus
   c. crux
   d. groove

350. The chordae tendineae may be categorized by all of the following terms except:
   a. primary
   b. secondary
   c. tertiary
   d. quarterly

351. All of the following cardiac valves normally have three leaflets except the:
   a. aortic
   b. mitral
   c. tricuspid
   d. pulmonic

352. The position of the heart in a tall, thin patient may be more:
   a. horizontal
   b. vertical
   c. lateral
   d. cephalad

353. The long axis of the heart is parallel to a line drawn from the:
    a. right shoulder to left hip
    b. left shoulder to right hip
    c. sternum to xyphoid process
    d. right shoulder to left shoulder

354. The descending thoracic aorta begins just beyond the:
    a. coronary arteries
    b. innominate artery
    c. left common carotid artery
    d. left subclavian artery

355. In relation to the spine, the aorta normally lies:
    a. to the right
    b. to the left
    c. cephalad
    d. inferior

356. The weakest area of the aorta is considered to be the aortic:
    a. annulus
    b. arch
    c. isthmus
    d. transverse

357. Which coronary artery is usually the dominant artery?
    a. left
    b. right
    c. left anterior descending
    d. circumflex

358. The left anterior descending coronary artery follows the:
    a. coronary sulcus
    b. interventricular groove
    c. atrioventricular groove
    d. coronary sinus

359. The left circumflex coronary artery follows the:
    a. coronary sulcus
    b. interventricular groove
    c. atrioventricular groove
    d. coronary sinus

APPENDIX C

360. The veins that join to form the superior vena cava are the:
    a.   innominate
    b.   carotid
    c.   internal
    d.   external

361. As compared to intrathoracic pressure, intrapericardial pressure is:
    a.   greater than
    b.   equal to
    c.   less than
    d.   cannot be predicted

362. All of the following are considered conotruncal abnormalities except:
    a.   truncus arteriosus
    b.   ventricular septal defect
    c.   tetralogy of Fallot
    d.   d-transposition of the great arteries

363. Depolarization of the ventricles occurs with the onset of the:
    a.   QRS complex
    b.   P wave
    c.   T wave
    d.   S wave

364. As compared to the beginning of left ventricular contraction, right ventricular contraction begins:
    a.   before
    b.   at the same time
    c.   after
    d.   varies

365. The period of time where the cardiac cell will not respond to another stimulus no matter how strong is called:
    a.   absolute refractory period
    b.   relative refractory period
    c.   rapid repolarization
    d.   partial repolarization

366. Which of the following states that the greater the stretch of the cardiac muscle cell, the greater the force of contraction.
    a.   Bernoulli
    b.   Doppler
    c.   Gorlin
    d.   Starling

367. The length to which a cardiac myofibril is stretched prior to the next contraction is called:
    a. afterload
    b. diastasis
    c. preload
    d. systole

368. Within limits, what effect will an increase in preload have on contraction?
    a. increase
    b. decrease
    c. varied
    d. cannot be predicted

369. All of the following will increase preload except:
    a. atrioventricular valve regurgitation
    b. atrioventricular valve stenosis
    c. semilunar valve regurgitation
    d. septal defects

370. _____ is the resistance the ventricles faces as it ejects blood.
    a. afterload
    b. diastole
    c. preload
    d. systole

371. Normally an increase in afterload will have what effect on the rate of ventricular fiber shortening?
    a. increase
    b. decrease
    c. no change
    d. cannot be predicted

372. All of the following pathologies will increase afterload except:
    a. semilunar valve stenosis
    b. semilunar valve regurgitation
    c. supravalvular stenosis
    d. systemic/pulmonary hypertension

373. According to the interval-strength relationship, sinus bradycardia may have which effect on ventricular contraction?
    a. increase
    b. decrease
    c. no change
    d. cannot be predicted

374. What effect will the compensatory pause following a premature ventricular contraction have on an aortic stenosis peak velocity?
    a.   increase
    b.   decrease
    c.   no effect
    d.   cannot be predicted

375. The atrioventricular valves close when:
    a.   atrial pressure exceeds ventricular pressure
    b.   ventricular pressure exceeds atrial pressure
    c.   arterial pressure exceeds ventricular pressure
    d.   ventricular pressure exceeds arterial pressure

376. The atrioventricular valves open when:
    a.   atrial pressure exceeds ventricular pressure
    b.   arterial pressure exceeds ventricular pressure
    c.   ventricular pressure exceeds arterial pressure
    d.   ventricular pressure exceeds atrial pressure

377. Semilunar valve opening occurs when:
    a.   arterial pressure exceeds ventricular pressure
    b.   ventricular pressure exceeds arterial pressure
    c.   atrial pressure exceeds ventricular pressure
    d.   ventricular pressure exceeds atrial pressure

378. Semilunar valve closure occurs when:
    a.   arterial pressure exceeds ventricular pressure
    b.   ventricular pressure exceeds arterial pressure
    c.   ventricular pressure exceeds atrial pressure
    d.   atrial pressure exceeds ventricular pressure

379. The pre-ejection period refers to:
    a.   ventricular diastole
    b.   diastasis
    c.   isovolumic contraction
    d.   active relaxation

380. What effect will valvular aortic stenosis have on ventricular ejection time?
    a.   increase
    b.   decrease
    c.   no change
    d.   cannot be predicted

381. Stenotic valve gradients may increase due to an increase in:
    a. flow volume
    b. valve area
    c. respiration
    d. turbulence

382. Chest pain is associated with all of the following except:
    a. coronary artery disease
    b. pericarditis
    c. musculoskeletal
    d. ascites

383. Peripheral edema may be associated with all of the following except:
    a. right heart failure
    b. mitral valve prolapse
    c. peripheral venous insufficiency
    d. liver failure

384. The pericardial friction rub may indicate:
    a. cardiac tumor
    b. hypertrophic cardiomyopathy
    c. rheumatic fever
    d. pericarditis

385. The auscultatory finding for constrictive pericarditis is:
    a. loud S1
    b. opening snap
    c. pericardial knock
    d. S4

386. The heart can begin and maintain rhythmic activity without the aid of the nervous system. This is called:
    a. automaticity
    b. excitability
    c. conductivity
    d. contractility

387. The cardiac muscle can accept and respond to electrical impulses. This is referred to as:
    a. contractility
    b. conductivity
    c. excitability
    d. automaticity

388. A cardiac cell is able to transfer an electrical impulse to a neighboring cardiac cell. This is called:
   a. excitability
   b. contractlity
   c. automaticity
   d. conductivity

389. The heart responds to an electrical impulse by contracting. This is called:
   a. automaticity
   b. contractility
   c. conductivity
   d. excitability

390. All of the following maneuvers increase cardiac output except:
   a. passive leg raising
   b. supine to standing
   c. squatting
   d. standing to walking

391. All of the following will cause a systolic murmur except:
   a. atrioventricular valve regurgitation
   b. atrioventricular valve stenosis
   c. semilunar valve stenosis
   d. hypertrophic cardiomyopathy

392. All of the following will cause a diastolic murmur except:
   a. aortic regurgitation
   b. mitral stenosis
   c. aortic stenosis
   d. pulmonary regurgitation

393. The right heart delivers blood to all of the following except the:
   a. vena cava
   b. main pulmonary artery
   c. pulmonary capillaries
   d. pulmonary veins

394. The phonocardiogram below is demonstrating:
   a. mitral stenosis
   b. aortic stenosis
   c. aortic regurgitation
   d. patent ductus arteriosus

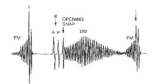

395. The phonocardiogram shown below is demonstrating:
    a.   mitral stenosis
    b.   aortic stenosis
    c.   hypertrophic cardiomyopathy
    d.   patent ductus arteriosus

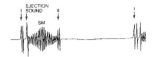

396. The phonocardiogram shown below is demonstrating:
    a.   mitral stenosis
    b.   aortic stenosis
    c.   aortic regurgitation
    d.   hypertrophic cardiomyopathy

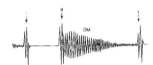

397. The phonocardiogram shown below is demonstrating:
    a.   hypertrophic cardiomyopathy
    b.   mitral regurgitation
    c.   mitral stenosis
    d.   patent ductus arteriosus

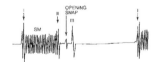

398. The phonocardiogram shown below is demonstrating:
    a.   heart sounds
    b.   heart murmurs
    c.   blood flow
    d.   jugular pulse

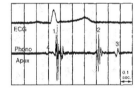

399. The electrocardiogram shown below is demonstrating:
    a.   normal sinus rhythm
    b.   sinus bradycardia
    c.   sinus tachycardia
    d.   atrial flutter

APPENDIX C

400. The electrocardiogram shown below is demonstrating:
    a.   normal sinus rhythm
    b.   sinus bradycardia
    c.   sinus tachycardia
    d.   sinus arrhythmia

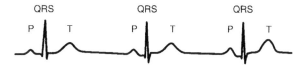

401. The electrocardiogram shown below is demonstrating:
    a.   normal sinus rhythm
    b.   sinus bradycardia
    c.   sinus tachycardia
    d.   sinus arrhythmia

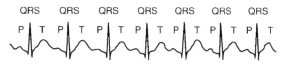

402. The electrocardiogram shown below is demonstrating:
    a.   normal sinus rhythm
    b.   sinus arrhythmia
    c.   sinus arrest
    d.   premature atrial contraction

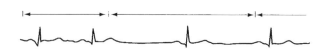

403. The electrocardiogram shown below is demonstrating:
    a.   normal sinus rhythm
    b.   sinus arrhythmia
    c.   sinus arrest
    d.   premature atrial contraction

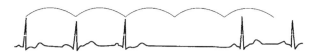

404. The electrocardiogram shown below is demonstrating:
    a.   normal sinus rhythm
    b.   sinus arrhythmia
    c.   sinus arrest
    d.   premature atrial contraction

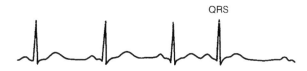

APPENDIX C

405. The electrocardiogram shown below is demonstrating:
  a. normal sinus rhythm
  b. atrial flutter
  c. atrial fibrillation
  d. premature ventricular contraction

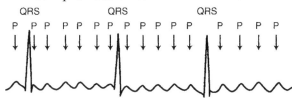

406. The electrocardiogram shown below is demonstrating:
  a. normal sinus rhythm
  b. atrial flutter
  c. atrial fibrillation
  d. premature ventricular contraction

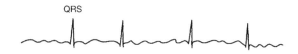

407. The electrocardiogram shown below is demonstrating:
  a. normal sinus rhythm
  b. atrial flutter
  c. atrial fibrillation
  d. premature ventricular contraction

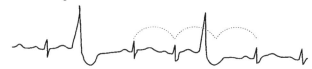

408. The electrocardiogram shown below is demonstrating:
  a. normal sinus rhythm
  b. ventricular tachycardia
  c. ventricular fibrillation
  d. first degree AV block

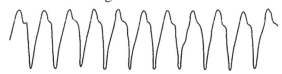

409. The electrocardiogram shown below is demonstrating:
  a. normal sinus ryhthm
  b. ventricular tachycardia
  c. ventricular fibrillation
  d. first degree AV block

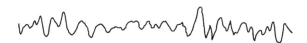

APPENDIX C

410. The electrocardiogram shown below is demonstrating:
   a. normal sinus rhythm
   b. ventricular tachycardia
   c. ventricular fibrillation
   d. first degree AV block

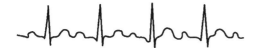

411. The electrocardiogram shown below is demonstrating:
   a. normal sinus rhythm
   b. second degree AV block
   c. third degree AV block
   d. artificial pacemaker

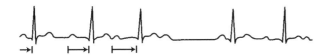

412. The electrocardiogram shown below is demonstrating:
   a. normal sinus rhythm
   b. second degree AV block
   c. third degree AV block
   d. artificial pacemaker

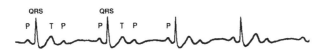

413. The electrocardiogram shown below is demonstrating:
   a. normal sinus rhythm
   b. second degree AV block
   c. third degree AV block
   d. artificial pacemaker

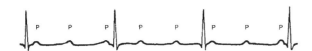

414. The cardiac catheterization pressure tracing shown below is demonstrating:
   a. normal
   b. aortic stenosis
   c. aortic regurgitation
   d. mitral stenosis

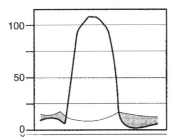

APPENDIX C

415. The cardiac catheterization pressure tracing shown below is demonstrating:
    a.   normal
    b.   aortic stenosis
    c.   pulmonic stenosis
    d.   mitral regurgitation

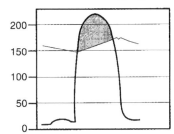

416. The cardiac catheterization pressure tracing shown below is demonstrating:
    a.   normal
    b.   aortic stenosis
    c.   pulmonic stenosis
    d.   mitral regurgitation

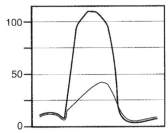

417. The cardiac catheterization pressure tracing shown below is demonstrating:
    a.   normal
    b.   aortic regurgitation
    c.   pulmonic regurgitation
    d.   mitral stenosis

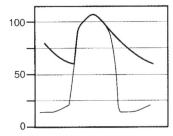

418. The cardiac catheterization pressure tracing shown below is demonstrating:
    a.   normal
    b.   aortic regurgitation
    c.   pulmonic regurgitation
    d.   mitral stenosis

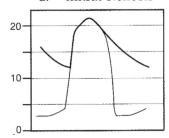

APPENDIX C

419. The cardiac catheterization pressure tracing shown below is demonstrating:
 a. normal
 b. mitral stenosis
 c. tricuspid stenosis
 d. aortic regurgitation

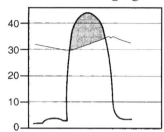

420. The cardiac catheterization pressure tracing shown below is demonstrating:
 a. normal
 b. mitral stenosis
 c. tricuspid stenosis
 d. pulmonic stenosis

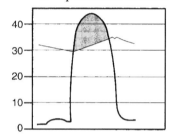

421. The cardiac catheterization pressure tracing shown below is demonstrating:
 a. normal
 b. mitral regurgitation
 c. tricuspid regurgitation
 d. aortic stenosis

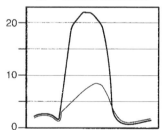

422. The tracing shown below is demonstrating:
 a. preload
 b. afterload
 c. myocardial contractility
 d. turbulence

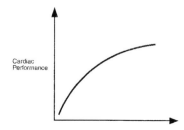

APPENDIX C

423. The tracing shown below is demonstrating:
   a. preload
   b. afterload
   c. myocardial contractility
   d. turbulence

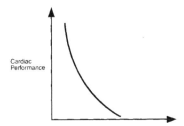

424. Ventricular systolic contraction begins at the:
   a. cardiac base
   b. cardiac apex
   c. lateral walls of the ventricles
   d. medial walls of the ventricles

425. In an uncomplicated atrial septal defect the shunt is predominantly:
   a. right to left
   b. left to right
   c. bidirectional
   d. cannot be predicted

426. Ventricular depolarization marks the beginning of ventricular:
   a. diastole
   b. diastasis
   c. systole
   d. relaxation

427. Ventricular repolarization represents ventricular:
   a. diastole
   b. diastasis
   c. systole
   d. contraction

428. According to the action potential curve for cardiac cells, actual cardiac contraction occurs during the electrocardiogram:
   a. P wave
   b. onset of the QRS complex
   c   ST segment
   d. PR interval

429. Normally which of the following cardiac chambers has the lowest pressure?
   a. right atrium
   b. left atrium
   c. right ventricle
   d. left ventricle

430. For valvular aortic stenosis which of the following is a true statement?
   a. increase in left ventricular systolic pressure, increase in aortic systolic pressure
   b. decrease in left ventricular systolic pressure, decrease in systolic aortic pressure
   c. increase in left ventricular systolic pressure, decrease in aortic systolic pressure
   d. decrease in left ventricular systolic pressure, increase in aortic systolic pressure

431. Which of the following is a true statement concerning mitral valve stenosis?
   a. increase in left atrial pressure, decrease in left ventricular diastolic pressure
   b. increase in left atrial pressure, increase in left ventricular diastolic pressure
   c. decrease in left atrial pressure, increase in left ventricular diastolic pressure
   d. decrease in left atrial pressure, decrease in left ventricular diastolic pressure

432. Which of the following pressures will most likely be increased in a patient with significant chronic aortic regurgitation?
   a. left atrial
   b. left ventricular end diastolic
   c. aortic diastolic
   d. pulmonary artery wedge

433. The PR interval is determined to be 223 milliseconds. The diagnosis is:
   a. first degree atrioventricular block
   b. Mobitz I
   c. Wenckebach
   d. complete heart block

434. While performing an echocardiogram the sonographer notes a structure in the right atrium. All of the following are possible explanations except:
   a. thebesian valve
   b. eustachian valve
   c. trabeculae carneae
   d. Chiari network

435. While observing a transesophageal examination the sonographer notes a structure in the left atrial appendage. The most likely anatomic explanation is that it is:
   a. trabeculae carneae
   b. pectinate muscle
   c. chordal web
   d. eustachian valve

APPENDIX C

436. During a venous saline contrast injection the patient performs a Valsalva maneuver and contrast crosses into the left atrium. The most likely explanation is:
    a. perimembranous ventricular septal defect
    b. left ventricle to right atrial communication
    c. patent foramen ovale
    d. partial anomalous pulmonary venous return

437. While performing an echocardiogram the sonographer notes a structure near the apex of the right ventricle. The most likely explanation is:
    a. chordal web
    b. moderator band
    c. pectinate muscle
    d. Chiari network

438. During a pediatric echocardiogram the sonographer is questioned on how to identify a right ventricle. All of the following are anatomical features of the right ventricle except:
    a. moderator band
    b. three papillary muscle groups
    c. smooth ventricular walls
    d. three leaflet atrioventricular valve

439. An echocardiogram request reads "Rule out infundibular stenosis." The sonographer should carefully evaluate the:
    a. left ventricular outflow tract
    b. right ventricular outflow tract
    c. left atrial appendage
    d. cardiac apex

440. An echocardiogram request reads "Rule out supracristal ventricular septal defect." The sonographer should carefully evaluate the:
    a. left ventricular outflow tract
    b. right ventricular outflow tract
    c. left atrial appendage
    d. cardiac apex

441. An echocardiogram request reads "Rule out left ventricular inflow tract obstruction." The sonographer should carefully evaluate all of the following except:
    a. valve annulus
    b. valve leaflets
    c. chordae tendineae
    d. trabeculae carneae

APPENDIX C

442. During an echocardiographic examination of a patient with long-standing severe pulmonary hypertension, the sonographer notes that the right ventricle forms the cardiac apex. This finding is anatomically:
   a. normal
   b. abnormal
   c. varies
   d. cannot be predicted

443. An echocardiogram request reads "Rule out perimembranous ventricular septal defect." The sonographer should carefully evaluate the:
   a. left ventricular outflow tract
   b. right ventricular outflow tract
   c. left atrial appendage
   d. cardiac apex

444. During an echocardiographic examination of a patient with long standing severe pulmonary hypertension the sonographer notes the interventricular septum is concave to the right ventricle. This finding is anatomically:
   a. normal
   b. abnormal
   c. varies
   d. cannot be predicted

445. During an echocardiogram the sonographer is questioned on which tricuspid valve leaflet is the largest. The correct answer is the:
   a. anterior
   b. posterior
   c. medial
   d. septal

446. During an echocardiogram examination the sonographer is questioned on which tricuspid valve leaflet is inserted closer to the cardiac apex. The correct response is:
   a. anterior
   b. posterior
   c. septal
   d. lateral

447. During a color flow Doppler examination the sonographer notes a moderate size mosaic backflow of blood into the right atrium during ventricular systole. This finding is called atrioventricular valve:
   a. stenosis
   b. regurgitation
   c. obstruction
   d. dissection

APPENDIX C

448. In the parasternal short-axis view of the mitral valve the sonographer may be able to evaluate all of the following except:
    a. anterior leaflet
    b. medial commissure
    c. lateral commissure
    d. septal leaflet

449. During a transesophageal examination the sonographer notes prominent echoes at the edges of each aortic valve cusp. A possible anatomic explanation would be:
    a. vestigial valve
    b. nodules of Arantii
    c. nodules of Atlantii
    d. ectopic chordae

450. In the standard parasternal long-axis view the sonographer may be able to evaluate all of the following sections of the aorta except the:
    a. aortic annulus
    b. transverse aorta
    c. sinotubular junction
    d. descending thoracic aorta

451. In the suprasternal long axis view the sonographer may be able to evaluate all of the following arteries except the:
    a. innominate
    b. left common carotid
    c. left subclavian
    d. superior mesenteric

452. An echocardiographic request reads "Rule out type III aortic dissection: question intimal tear at the aortic isthmus." The best two-dimensional view the sonographer may use to evaluate the aortic isthmus is the:
    a. parasternal long axis
    b. parasternal short axis of the aortic valve
    c. apical four chamber
    d. suprasternal long axis

453. An echocardiogram examination is ordered for a patient with known left anterior descending coronary artery disease. The sonographer should expect to see wall motion abnormalities in all of the following left ventricular wall segments except:
    a. anterior septum
    b. anterior
    c. anterolateral
    d. cardiac apex

APPENDIX C

454. An echocardiogram examination is ordered for a patient with known left circumflex coronary artery disease. The sonographer should expect to see wall motion abnormalities in all of the following left ventricular wall segments except:
    a. anterior septum
    b. anterolateral
    c. inferolateral
    d. lateral

455. During an echocardiographic examination the sonographer notes a segmental wall motion abnormality of the inferior interventricular septum. The coronary artery most likely causing this abnormality is the:
    a. left main
    b. left anterior descending
    c. left circumflex
    d. posterior descending

456. During an echocardiographic examination the sonographer notes a wall motion abnormality of the lateral wall of the right ventricle. The coronary artery most likely diseased is the:
    a. left main
    b. oblique margin
    c. diagonal
    d. acute margin

457. In the parasternal long axis view the sonographer notes an echo free space at the roof of the left atrium. The most likely anatomic explanation is that it is the:
    a. aortic sinotubular junction
    b. atrial appendage
    c. oblique sinus
    d. left pulmonary artery

458. During a color flow Doppler examination the sonographer notes flow into the right atrium. All of the following are possible explanations except:
    a. superior vena cava flow
    b. inferior vena cava flow
    c. coronary sinus flow
    d. ductus venosus flow

459. During a left heart contrast echocardiographic examination, flow is noted in the left ventricle during ventricular diastole. All of the following are possible explanations except:
    a. mitral valve inflow
    b. aortic regurgitation
    c. thebesian venous flow
    d. atrial septal defect flow

460. During an echocardiographic examination the sonographer notes an anterior clear space located between the epicardium and myocardium. The most likely explanation is:
   a. pericardial effusion
   b. adipose tissue
   c. pleural effusion
   d. dilated coronary sinus

461. During an echocardiographic examination the sonographer notes pericardial effusion behind the left atrium. This effusion is contained in the:
   a. transverse sinus
   b. oblique sinus
   c. coronary sinus
   d. sinus of Valsalva

462. During a transesophageal examination, the sonographer notes a clear space between the pulmonary artery and the aorta. This is most likely the:
   a. transverse sinus
   b. oblique sinus
   c. coronary sinus
   d. carotid sinus

463. While evaluating left ventricular systolic function in the apical four chamber view, the sonographer should expect the base of the heart to move:
   a. posteriorly
   b. laterally
   c. downward
   d. caudad

464. In the parasternal short axis view of the cardiac apex, the sonographer should normally expect to visualize the heart to twist:
   a. clockwise
   b. counterclockwise
   c. posteriorly
   d. laterally

465. During an echocardiographic evaluation of a patient with severe, acute aortic regurgitation the sonographer notes premature closure of the mitral valve. The most likely explanantion is that there is an increase in:
   a. left atrial pressure
   b. left ventricular end diastolic pressure
   c. aortic pressure
   d. heart rate

APPENDIX C

466. During an echocardiographic examination of a patient with constrictive pericarditis the sonographer notes premature opening of the pulmonic valve. The most likely explanation is that there is an increase in:
    a. right atrial pressure
    b. right ventricular end-diastolic pressure
    c. pulmonary artery pressure
    d. heart rate

467. During an echocardiographic examination of a patient with a history of systemic hypertension the sonographer measures and notes an abnormal increase in the time interval between aortic valve closure and mitral valve opening. This represents an abnormality during:
    a. early ventricular systole
    b. early ventricular diastole
    c. diastasis
    d. pre-ejection period

468. During an echocardiographic examination of a patient with dilated cardiomyopathy the sonographer notes an abnormal increase in the time period between mitral valve closure and aortic valve opening. This represents an abnormality during:
    a. early ventricular diastole
    b. late ventricular systole
    c. diastasis
    d. pre-ejection period

469. The sonographer measures a left ventricular end diastolic volume of 120 cc and an left ventricular end systolic volume of 90 cc. The heart rate is 80 beats per minute. The body surface area is 2.0 m^2. The stroke volume in this case is:
    a. increased
    b. normal
    c. abnormal
    d. cannot be predicted

470. The sonographer measures a left ventricular end diastolic volume of 100 cc and a left ventricular systolic volume of 30 cc. The heart rate is 50 beats per minute. The body surface area is 2.0 m^2. The cardiac output is:
    a. 30 cc
    b. 130 cc
    c. 3500 cc
    d. 6500 cc

471. The sonographer measures a left ventricular end diastolic volume of 120 cc and a left ventricular end systolic volume of 60 cc. The heart rate is 70 beats per minute. The body surface area is 2.0 m^2. The cardiac index is:
    a. 30 cc
    b. 1.1 lpm/m^2
    c. 2.1 lpm/m^2
    d. 4.2 lpm/m^2

APPENDIX C

472. The sonographer measures an end systolic volume of 40 cc and an end diastolic volume of 80 cc. The heart rate is 110 beats per minute. The body surface area is 1.8 m². The ejection fraction is:
    a. 40 cc
    b. 120 cc
    c. 33 %
    d. 50 %

473. A 22 year old female presents with the diagnosis of univentricular heart. The echocardiogram demonstrates a smooth walled ventricle. The ventricle is most likely a morphologic:
    a. right ventricle
    b. left ventricle
    c. combination right and left ventricle
    d. cannot be predicted

474. By evaluating the inferior vena cava the sonographer predicts the right atrial pressure to be 10 mm Hg. In the absence of right ventricular inflow tract obstruction, which other cardiac pressure is equal to 10 mm Hg?
    a. right ventricular diastolic
    b. right ventricular systolic
    c. pulmonary artery systolic
    d. pulmonary artery diastolic

475. Utilizing the tricuspid regurgitation method the sonographer predicts the right ventricular systolic pressure to be 65 mm Hg. In the absence of right ventricular outflow tract obstruction which other cardiac pressure would be 65 mm Hg?
    a. pulmonary artery diastolic
    b. pulmonary artery mean
    c. pulmonary artery systolic
    d. left atrial mean

476. Utilizing the pulmonary regurgitation method the sonographer predicts the pulmonary end diastolic pressure to be 19 mm Hg. What other cardiac pressures would be equal to 19 mm Hg?
    a. pulmonary artery systolic and mean
    b. right atrial and right ventricular end diastolic
    c. left atrial and left ventricular diastolic
    d. aortic systolic and diastolic

477. The sonographer determines a patient's blood pressure to be 133/76 mm Hg. In the absence of left ventricular outflow tract obstruction, which other cardiac chamber would have a systolic pressure of 133 mm Hg.
    a. pulmonary systolic
    b. left atrial
    c. left ventricle
    d. mean aortic

APPENDIX C

478. While reviewing a patient's cardiac catheterization report before performing an echocardiographic examination, the sonographer notes the right atrial v wave was measured to be 18 mm Hg. The expected cardiac Doppler finding would be significant:
    a. aortic regurgitation
    b. mitral regurgitation
    c. tricuspid regurgitation
    d. pulmonic regurgitation

479. While performing a continuous wave Doppler examination of a patient with hypertrophic obstructive cardiomyopathy the sonographer requests the patient perform a Valsalva maneuver. The velocity across the obstruction should:
    a. increase
    b. decrease
    c. unaffected
    d. cannot be predicted

480. While performing a continuous wave Doppler examination of a patient with known hypertrophic cardiomyopathy the sonographer administers amyl nitrite. The velocity across the obstruction should:
    a. increase
    b. decrease
    c. unaffected
    d. cannot be predicted

481. While performing a color flow Doppler examination of a patient with mitral regurgitation the sonographer requests the patient to perform an isometric handgrip. The effect on the mitral regurgitation jet size will be:
    a. increased
    b. decreased
    c. unaffected
    d. cannot be predicted

482. While reviewing a patient's chart before performing an echocardiogram, the sonographer notes that the physician heard a decrease in the systolic murmur while the patient went from a standing position to a squatting position. The sonographer should expect:
    a. valvular aortic stenosis
    b. mitral valve stenosis
    c. tricuspid regurgitation
    d. hypertrophic obstructive cardiomyopathy

483. Before performing an echocardiogram the sonographer reviews the patient's chart which states the physician heard a loud S1, opening snap and late diastolic murmur. The sonographer should expect to see:
    a. mitral valve prolapse
    b. valvular aortic stenosis
    c. rheumatic mitral stenosis
    d. aortic regurgitation

APPENDIX C

484. Before performing an echocardiogram the sonographer reviews the patient's chart, which states the physician heard a crescendo-decrescendo systolic ejection murmur at the right upper sternal border and an S4. The sonographer should expect to see:
    a. mitral valve prolapse
    b. valvular aortic stenosis
    c. rheumatic mitral stenosis
    d. mitral regurgitation

485. Before performing an echocardiogram the sonographer reviews the patient's, chart which states the physician heard a mid-systolic click and a late systolic murmur at the cardiac apex. The sonographer should expect to see:
    a. mitral valve prolapse
    b. valvular aortic stenosis
    c. rheumatic mitral stenosis
    d. aortic regurgitation

486. Before performing an echocardiogram the sonographer reviews the patient's chart which states the physician heard a holosystolic murmur at the xyphoid region that increased with inspiration. The sonographer should expect to see:
    a. aortic regurgitation
    b. mitral regurgitation
    c. tricuspid regurgitation
    d. pulmonic regurgitation

487. Before performing an echocardiogram the sonographer reviews the patient's chart, which states the physician heard a pansystolic murmur and an S3 at the cardiac apex. The sonographer should expect to see:
    a. aortic regurgitation
    b. mitral regurgitation
    c. mitral stenosis
    d. pulmonic regurgitation

488. Before beginning an echocardiogram the sonographer reviews the patient's chart which states the patient's main complaint is sudden shortness of breath at night. The sonographer should expect to find (a):
    a. normal heart
    b. left ventricular failure
    c. cardiac arryhthmia
    d. acute myocardial infarction

489. Before performing an echocardiogram the sonographer reviews the patient's chart which states that the patient presented with syncope. The sonographer should be careful to rule out:
    a. pericarditis
    b. pleural effusion
    c. dilated cardiomyopathy
    d. valvular aortic stenosis

APPENDIX C

490. Before beginning an echocardiogram the sonographer reviews the patient's chart and finds that the right atrial pressure was increased at cardiac catheterization. All of the following are possible reasons except:
    a. tricuspid stenosis
    b. right ventricular infarction
    c. decreased circulating blood volume
    d. pulmonary hypertension

491. The sonographer reviews a patient's chart before beginning an echocardiogram and notes that the patient has increased pulmonary artery pressures. All of the following may be possible explanations except:
    a. pericardial effusion
    b. mitral stenosis
    c. left ventricular failure
    d. left to right cardiac shunt

492. The sonographer notes the pulmonary artery wedge pressure to be 16 mm Hg. This pressure reflects the left ventricular end diastolic pressure in all of the following pathologies except:
    a. mitral regurgitation
    b. mitral stenosis
    c. cardiac tamponade
    d. systemic hypertension

493. The sonographer reviews the patient's chart before starting the echocardiogram and notes that the pulmonary artery wedge pressure is abnormally low. The best possible explanation would be:
    a. mitral stenosis
    b. left ventricular failure
    c. cardiac amyloidosis
    d. hypovolemia

494. Before performing an echocardiogram the sonographer reviews the patient's chest x-ray report that states the patient has cardiomegaly. Based on this finding the sonographer may see:
    a. constrictive pericarditis
    b. pericardial effusion
    c. aortic aneurysm
    d. normal heart

495. During an echocardiographic examination the nuclear cardiology laboratory requests the sonographer to bring the patient for a MUGA. The most likely reason for the MUGA test is:
    a. visualize myocardial perfusion
    b. visualize coronary artery blood flow
    c. evaluate ejection fraction
    d. evaluate physiologic heart function

APPENDIX C

496. Before beginning an echocardiogram, the sonographer reviews a patient's cardiac catheterization and finds the patient has giant right atrial a waves. The sonographer may find:
    a. tricuspid stenosis
    b. mitral stenosis
    c. left heart failure
    d. tricuspid regurgitation

497. During a continuous wave Doppler examination of tricuspid regurgitation the sonographer notes a peak velocity of 3.3 m/s. The pressure gradient between the right atrium and right ventricle during ventricular systole is:
    a. increased
    b. decreased
    c. normal
    d. cannot be predicted

498. During a continuous wave Doppler examination of mitral regurgitation, the sonographer notes a peak velocity of 5.0 m/s. The pressure gradient between the left atrium and left ventricle during ventricular systole is:
    a. normal
    b. increased
    c. decreased
    d. cannot be predicted

499. During a continuous wave Doppler examination of the aortic valve the sonographer notes a peak velocity of 4.0 m/s. The peak velocity across the left ventricular outflow tract is 2.0 m/s. The peak pressure gradient across the aortic valve is:
    a. 4 mm Hg
    b. 16 mm Hg
    c. 48 mm Hg
    d. 64 mm Hg

500. During a pulsed wave Doppler examination of the pulmonary veins the sonographer notes giant atrial reversal waves. The most likely explanation is:
    a. mitral regurgitation
    b. aortic stenosis
    c. increased left ventricular end diastolic pressure
    d. hypovolemia

APPENDIX C

THE CARDIOVASCULAR PRINCIPLES 500

1. b	51. c	101. b	151. d
2. c	52. a	102. d	152. c
3. d	53. c	103. a	153. c
4. d	54. b	104. a	154. a
5. b	55. b	105. b	155. d
6. a	56. c	106. b	156. c
7. d	57. b	107. b	157. b
8. b	58. a	108. d	158. d
9. c	59. d	109. c	159. b
10. b	60. b	110. b	160. a
11. b	61. a	111. d	161. a
12. d	62. a	112. a	162. b
13. c	63. c	113. b	163. b
14. d	64. c	114. c	164. a
15. a	65. c	115. a	165. c
16. c	66. d	116. b	166. a
17. d	67. a	117. d	167. d
18. c	68. c	118. c	168. a
19. c	69. a	119. b	169. b
20. b	70. a	120. d	170. a
21. c	71. c	121. a	171. d
22. d	72. b	122. c	172. b
23. d	73. d	123. b	173. d
24. d	74. c	124. c	174. a
25. d	75. a	125. a	175. b
26. c	76. b	126. c	176. b
27. d	77. b	127. b	177. c
28. a	78. c	128. c	178. b
29. c	79. c	129. c	179. c
30. a	80. b	130. d	180. b
31. b	81. b	131. d	181. d
32. c	82. c	132. b	182. b
33. b	83. d	133. c	183. b
34. c	84. c	134. c	184. a
35. c	85. c	135. d	185. a
36. c	86. c	136. d	186. c
37. b	87. c	137. a	187. c
38. b	88. a	138. b	188. c
39. d	89. d	139. c	189. a
40. c	90. a	140. d	190. a
41. a	91. d	141. a	191. d
42. c	92. a	142. b	192. c
43. b	93. b	143. c	193. d
44. c	94. d	144. d	194. a
45. c	95. c	145. a	195. d
46. d	96. a	146. d	196. b
47. c	97. b	147. d	197. d
48. b	98. a	148. d	198. d
49. d	99. d	149. d	199. a
50. b	100. d	150. d	200. a

APPENDIX C

201. c	251. d	301. d	351. b
202. b	252. d	302. c	352. b
203. a	253. c	303. b	353. a
204. d	254. a	304. d	354. d
205. b	255. b	305. b	355. b
206. a	256. b	306. d	356. c
207. b	257. a	307. c	357. b
208. c	258. b	308. a	358. b
209. c	259. c	309. b	359. c
210. b	260. d	310. c	360. a
211. d	261. c	311. a	361. b
212. b	262. d	312. b	362. b
213. d	263. a	313. b	363. a
214. c	264. b	314. d	364. c
215. c	265. c	315. a	365. a
216. b	266. b	316. a	366. d
217. d	267. d	317. b	367. c
218. a	268. b	318. b	368. a
219. c	269. c	319. b	369. b
220. c	270. d	320. a	370. a
221. c	271. a	321. a	371. b
222. a	272. b	322. b	372. b
223. a	273. d	323. d	373. a
224. c	274. d	324. c	374. a
225. b	275. d	325. c	375. b
226. a	276. a	326. b	376. a
227. c	277. c	327. b	377. b
228. c	278. a	328. c	378. a
229. c	279. a	329. d	379. c
230. c	280. c	330. c	380. a
231. a	281. c	331. a	381. a
232. b	282. a	332. b	382. d
233. b	283. d	333. b	383. b
234. c	284. a	334. a	384. d
235. a	285. d	335. a	385. c
236. d	286. a	336. a	386. a
237. b	287. b	337. a	387. c
238. a	288. c	338. c	388. d
239. a	289. c	339. b	389. b
240. c	290. c	340. a	390. a
241. a	291. c	341. a	391. b
242. d	292. b	342. c	392. c
243. d	293. d	343. b	393. a
244. c	294. c	344. a	394. a
245. d	295. b	345. b	395. b
246. d	296. b	346. b	396. c
247. b	297. b	347. b	397. b
248. c	298. c	348. c	398. a
249. c	299. d	349. c	399. a
250. b	300. a	350. d	400. b

APPENDIX C

401. c
402. b
403. c
404. d
405. b
406. c
407. d
408. b
409. c
410. d
411. b
412. b
413. c
414. d
415. b
416. d
417. b
418. c
419. c
420. d
421. c
422. a
423. b
424. b
425. b
426. c
427. a
428. c
429. a
430. c
431. a
432. b
433. a
434. c
435. b
436. c
437. b
438. c
439. b
440. b
441. d
442. b
443. a
444. b
445. a
446. c
447. b
448. d
449. b
450. b

451. d
452. d
453. c
454. a
455. d
456. d
457. d
458. d
459. d
460. b
461. b
462. a
463. c
464. b
465. b
466. b
467. b
468. d
469. c
470. c
471. c
472. d
473. b
474. a
475. c
476. c
477. c
478. c
479. a
480. a
481. a
482. d
483. c
484. b
485. a
486. c
487. b
488. b
489. d
490. c
491. a
492. b
493. d
494. b
495. c
496. a
497. a
498. a
499. c
500. c

APPENDIX C

APPENDIX D. ULTRASOUND SOCIETIES

AMERICAN INSTITUTE OF ULTRASOUND IN MEDICINE(AIUM)
14750 Sweitzer Lane, Suite 100
Laurel, Maryland 20707
(301) 498-4100
www.aium.org

AMERICAN REGISTRY FOR DIAGNOSTIC MEDICAL SONOGRAPHERS (ARDMS)
51 Monroe Street, Plaza East 1
Rockville, Maryland 20850
(301) 738-8401 or (800) 541-9754
www.ardms.org

AMERICAN SOCIETY OF ECHOCARDIOGRAPHY (ASE)
1500 Sunday Dr, Suite 102
Raleigh, North Carolina 27607
(919) 787-5181
www.asecho.org

CANADIAN SOCIETY OF DIAGNOSTIC MEDICAL SONOGRAPHERS (CSMDS)
PO BOX 1220
Kempville, ON
KOG1JO
888-273-6746
www.csdms.com

CARDIOVASCULAR CREDENTIALING INTERNATIONAL (CCI)
1500 Sunday Dr, Suite 102
Raleigh, North Carolina 27607
(919) 861-4539 or (800) 326-0268
www.cci-online.org

SOCIETY OF DIAGNOSTIC MEDICAL SONOGRAPHERS (SDMS)
2745 N. Dallas Parkway, Suite 350
Plano, Texas 75093
(800) 229-9506
www.sdms.org

SOCIETY OF VASCULAR ULTRASOUND (SVU)
4601 Presidents Drive, Suite 260
Lanham, Maryland 20706
(301) 459-7550
www.svunet.org

APPENDIX D